Acknowledgments

I would like to thank my family, friends, and patients who have con-
fided, guided, and decided to share their personal stories with me over
the years. The insight, support, and love from my close family (all
of you) have provided me with strength and wisdom. Thanks, Mom
and Dad, for showing me how a great relationship is supposed to go
down. A special thanks to Dr. Morgan for being such a great friend
and for teaching me so much. Barb, you're awesome.

Dr. Fleisher

I dedicate this book to my daughters Cara and Sam for their ever-con-
stant encouragement and love—and to my dear friend, Dr. Robert
Fleisher. Appreciation goes to my patients who trusted me enough
to courageously tell me about their sexless marriages and feelings of
loss. Quite often, patients are my greatest teachers as they teach me
what I don't know and what I need to study and learn.

Dr. Morgan

Dr. Fleisher and Dr. Morgan would like to express deepest appreciation for the brilliant performance of editor Bobby Waddell who
had the complex task of organizing this material. Her outstanding
effort helped produce a most important work to help couples remain
connected. Great appreciation and credit also go to our publisher
Norman Goldfind who had the vision, foresight, and courage to take
on this project.

RESCUING A SEXLESS MARRIAGE AND
MAKING IT ALL IT CAN BE USING THIS
EMPOWERING INTEGRATIVE APPROACH

the sexless marriage *fix*

Robert M. Fleisher, D.M.D.
Roberta Foss-Morgan, D.O.

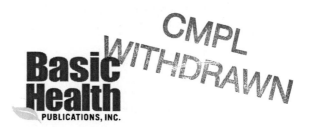

Basic Health
PUBLICATIONS, INC.

Basic Health Publications, Inc.
an imprint of
Turner Publishing Company
424 Church Street • Suite 2240 • Nashville, Tennessee 37219
445 Park Avenue • 9th Floor • New York, New York 10022
www.turnerpublishing.com

The Sexless Marriage Fix

The information contained in this book is based upon the research and personal and professional experiences of the authors. It is not intended as a substitute for consulting with your physician or other healthcare provider. Any attempt to diagnose and treat an illness should be done under the direction of a healthcare professional.

The publisher does not advocate the use of any particular healthcare protocol but believes the information in this book should be available to the public. The publisher and authors are not responsible for any adverse effects or consequences resulting from the use of the suggestions, preparations, or procedures discussed in this book. Should the reader have any questions concerning the appropriateness of any procedures or preparation mentioned, the authors and the publisher strongly suggest consulting a professional healthcare advisor.

Library of Congress Cataloging-in-Publication Data is available through the Library of Congress

Editor: Roberta W. Waddell
Typesetting/Book design: Gary A. Rosenberg
Cover design: Mike Stromberg

Printed in the United States of America
10 9 8 7 6 5 4 3 2 1

Contents

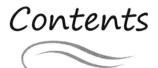

Please note that the book has been written by two doctors. To distinguish between them, (RM) will be used when Dr. Roberta Morgan is being quoted, and (RF) will be used when Dr. Robert Fleisher is being quoted.

Foreword

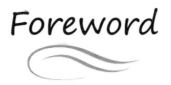

RALPH GOLAN, M.D.

The Sexless Marriage—How to Fix It, How to Prevent It by Dr. Morgan and Dr. Fleisher is a most welcome, excellent, and unusual addition to the self-help literature on improving marriage (or other primary relationships). What makes the book unusual is that it not only reviews the psychological/emotional/social reasons for how couples drift apart, but also discusses how medical, physiological, and hormonal changes impact the way couples relate, most particularly as they age.

What you will learn from this book is most likely what your primary care or family doctor cannot teach you—nor can your gynecologist, urologist, endocrinologist, therapist, or marriage counselor. You may learn vital information from each of these specialists certainly, but it would be rare that you would be given the whole picture and a clear path on how to proceed. The integrative-medicine approach found in this book connects all of these specialties into a practical, no-nonsense guide that may not only save your marriage, but could also improve your health immeasurably: your energy, sleep, and cognitive function, your mood, your weight, your heart, your bone density, your libido, and more . . .

Dr. Golan is an integrative-medicine practitioner in Seattle, WA, and the author of *Optimal Wellness: Where Mainstream and Alternative Medicine Meet.*

Dr. Morgan and Dr. Fleisher write in a manner that is friendly, nonjudgmental, interlaced with humor, and at the same time authoritative. They know human nature and the human body. They can now help you. This book is a gift that will empower you to take back control of your life.

1

The Nutshell

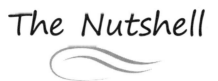

Most people don't think about a sexless marriage until they find themselves involved in one. It can creep up on you because, for most, the frequency of sex and the nature of sexual relationships changes over time, and if couples aren't careful, relationships can go into decline. In a nutshell, there are six causes of the sexless marriage. With your participation they can be fixed. Here we go.

Personal Issues

Personal issues, including lost love, boredom, changes in interests, financial woes, and others, need to be addressed with the understanding that dissolution of the marriage may be a choice if those involved are unable to find a resolution. Some avoid confronting personal issues due to fear, embarrassment, financial reasons, or inability to engage in the conversation. The help of a therapist may be needed in these cases. It is not easy to put the ego on the shelf, listen, and be willing to change. Marriage is for grownups, and working through problems is for those who are committed to making it work.

Behavioral Issues

These include neglecting your partner, withholding sex, nagging, negativity, not listening, loss of affection and kindness, and infidelity, and they all have to do with deeds or conduct that is not conducive to healthy relationships. If these behaviors are not remedied and continue without resolution, the relationship will yield unhealthy and,

1

at times, unbearable feelings, and become dysfunctional, or lead to outright failure.

Physical Issues

Physical erectile dysfunction, painful sex, incontinence, heart problems, or other medical problems need to be addressed by the appropriate healthcare providers. If the physical issues are sexual in nature, a gynecologist and/or urologist need to be consulted.

Psychological Issues

Depression, frigidity, *psychological* erectile dysfunction, and others, need to be addressed with therapy by a marriage counselor, psychologist, psychiatrist, family physician, or clergy. Counseling, and sometimes medication, helps resolve the psychological issues carried in locked suitcases to the honeymoon suite.

Hormonal Issues

Hormones affect many aspects of sexuality, as well as physical and psychological well-being, and issues involving them need to be addressed by a doctor trained and knowledgeable in hormonal replacement and human sexuality. But it's not just any kind of hormone replacement, with conventional, unsafe prescription medications. As will be discussed, there is a big difference between patent pharmaceuticals and *compounded bio-identical hormones*.

Combination Issues

Very likely, a sexless marriage is the result of more than one problem. It is often a combination of several issues that require the talents of the therapist and/or physician combined with desire and hard work on the part of the couple involved.

This combination of causes can make diagnosis and getting better a challenge. Receiving the appropriate care is something that requires your participation and your understanding of all the potential causes, so you know what to do and where to go for proper healing.

The Problem

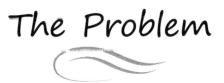

Do You Have a Problem?

THE DIVORCE RATE HAS BEEN RISING. TRADITIONAL VALUES AND behaviors have changed radically. People are no longer willing to stay in destructive or unhappy relationships. Perhaps due to society's emphasis on immediate gratification, they often don't take the steps required to improve the situation.

It is important to understand that some sexless marriages will fail if both partners are not on board with finding a solution. Depending on the cause or causes of the problem, there may be a simple solution. But, because the *fix* is not always easy, the cure is not for everyone. On the other hand though, perhaps frustration can become the opportunity to reinvent the joy you found in each other at one time.

It's Often Not Just One Thing That's Wrong

The sexless marriage is not usually the result of one issue. There are many reasons that relationships become sexless. Your particular situation is unique to you and your mate. You have to figure out what ails your relationship by giving it some deep thought.

If you are depressed, taking an antidepressant may help if the medication fixes a chemical imbalance that is the root cause, but what if the root cause for the depression is feeling unloved by an inattentive mate? *Your* medication is not going to get your mate to be more attentive. Maybe it's time to look for the cause of his/her inattentiveness. Are you no longer desirable to your mate? Could your mate feel that you no longer desire him/her? Are there stressors on the relationship, such as financial problems, illness, or grief? Is it lost libido that resulted from a hormonal decline on either you or your partner's part? Or is there another man/woman?

To better understand the interconnection between destructive factors in a sexual relationship, consider that if your mate's libido is shot as a result of low hormone levels, the replacement of these hormones may fix his/her libido, his/her inattentiveness, and *your* depression. That's a whole lot of bang for the buck and you may have never needed that antidepressant prescription after all.

What is Sexless?

Some experts define a sexless marriage as having sex ten or fewer times a year.[1] You may suddenly realize you're in a sexless marriage. Many of those in sexless marriages vehemently disagree and say it's the quality that counts. Actually, the frequency of sex is also an important parameter of marital communion and quality of life.

Frequency does vary by age. If a ninety-year-old couple is having sex five times a year, that's pretty phenomenal. It's not sexless, it's just *less sex*. However, if a twenty-five-year-old couple is having sex five times a year, there's probably something wrong, unless they both have no interest in sex. We could label that a happy sexless marriage.

To judge how good your sex life really is, it makes sense to compare yourself to others in your situation. Of course, it's not easy to go around asking your friends and contemporaries how often they *do it*. Pretty soon you won't have any friends. Most people don't talk about sex, even to their physicians or therapists.

If you did ask others about their sexual frequency, many would be embarrassed to tell the truth. To get the *real* story, we contacted Tom W. Smith, author of *American Sexual Behavior,* from the National Opinion Research Center (NORC) at the University of Chicago, and the information he provided was enlightening.[2]

On average, **all** *adults engage in sex about 60 times a year.* In the forties, the average is 64 times a year; by the fifties it's 47.4 times a year, almost once a week. Depending upon how you compare to these averages, you may start feeling pretty good, or you may start to badger your mate for more frequent encounters. These averages are for married and unmarried folks. Married couples are having more sex *on average* than singles because they live with a partner, thus making sexual encounters more available than for those who live alone. The yearly figures for married vs. not married are:

- 69.2 vs. 49.8 times a year in the forties;
- 53.8 vs. 31.2 times a year in the fifties;
- 32.5 vs. 15.7 times a year in the sixties;
- And 16.2 vs. 2.6 times a year in the seventies.

So if you thought singles-scene folks do it every night, guess again. Still, according to the above figures, if you're married, you're supposed to be doing it around once a week in your fifties.

Note that for couples in their sixties, sexual encounters go down to 32.5 times a year, and in the seventies, the frequency drops to 16.2 times a year. That's once a month—each birthday, New Years Eve if you don't get drunk and fall asleep, and once on Groundhog Day. Bear in mind that these are averages, and for many couples the frequency of sex is much less. According to some expert opinions, many couples are already living sexless lives.

While these statistics are stunning, the reasons for sexual decline are probably more compelling. Why does sexual frequency wane as people age? Why do so many people stop having sex altogether as they age? Is it natural to decrease the frequency and ultimately stop having sex? It all depends on how you define natural. The body ages, hormones are in decline, and various maladies develop. You can argue that decline is *the natural order of things,* or you can argue that there are remedies to fix many of the problems associated with aging and the decline of sexual activity, so why not use them?

The Natural Order of Things

Based on this natural order of things, sexual ability can extend from around the beginning of puberty (10–14 years of age)[3] to the later stages of life (the eighties), though this is the *range* and by no means the average. More likely, you can expect to have high-quality sex from the late teens to the late fifties. These numbers change from society to society and from era to era. In certain cultures today, children engage in sexual activity before the teen years, and these same cultures often see the age span reduced due to shortened life expectancy.

Why is Marriage Being Rejected?

There are three reasons why so many people are unmarried. They've never been married, there's a divorce, or the death of a spouse. In recent times, divorced and never-married statistics have skyrocketed, partly because it has never been easier. Gone is the stigma associated with those who never marry or remarry, and the taboos associated with divorce are no longer the force they were years ago.

Many of those divorcing or becoming widows/widowers never find a new mate, some by choice and others by circumstance. Some, after having had the experience of marriage, realize they are more content being single. Some bemoan the fact that they could never replace their perfect mate, and some were part of a dysfunctional family and do not wish to chance repeating such an experience.

It is common that people get divorced due to sexual incompatibilities.[4] People having great and frequent sex with their partners don't usually part ways unless other divisive reasons exist. The reasons for sexual decline and increasing numbers of single people often go deeper. Those with sexual dysfunctions that remain unresolved may often choose to remain alone.

Of course, incompatibilities are not just sexual. There are a host of important intellectual, emotional, and spiritual qualities that may not be evident during *courtship lust*. While these disconnects are also responsible for divorce, this book is predominately concerned with sexual issues.

Your Husband Wants Sex, Not a Baby

(RM) Women complain to me about how awful they feel. They state that they have hot flashes, night sweats, and debilitating insomnia, which all result in fatigue. They are taking a sleeping pill but it isn't working.

Wait, there's much more. They say that their moods are unstable and they are experiencing new onset anxiety and depression. They are seeing a psychiatrist and taking a tranquilizer and an antidepressant, which aren't helping either.

Their new weight set-point is ten to fifteen pounds heavier than it was a few years ago. According to theory, weight set-point is how much fat you can carry, a sort of thermostat for body fat. With women, it seems like they just woke up one morning with a muffin top and new layers of fat everywhere. To make it worse, this fat is resistant to the weight loss efforts that always worked in the past.

Their hair is thinning, brittle, dry and it is falling out by handfuls. Women have actually brought in baggies of hair to validate their predicament.

In the interview, I ask, "Do you still have a sex drive?" Then the floodgates open and tissues are dispensed in abundance.

They tell me, "Everything is dry and itchy, my hair, my skin, and my vagina. I'm always on an antibiotic for a urinary tract infection, and forget about sex. My vaginal dryness makes sex, which I previously enjoyed, such a wifely chore. Even if I use lubrication, it takes forever to reach orgasm, and then I have to ask myself if I really had one. There was a whimper of a feeling; at least I think there was. I used to feel a bang, not a whimper. Honestly doctor—I love my husband, but if something, God forbid, happened to him, I wouldn't date, and I wouldn't even masturbate. I feel dead from the waist down. I feel foggy on top and fat in the middle. Sex is honestly the very last thing on my mind."

Houston, We Have a Problem

Women are wise to learn that men need sex. Men usually communicate sexually, not verbally. Make a note to self—men will usually open energetically if they are having their sexual needs satisfied. Do a little experiment and have your doctor inject you with testosterone and you may have some idea of what men think about every 15 minutes. Meanwhile, women usually think about their weight every 15 minutes or so.

Doctors are not usually trained in sexology, nutrition, or weight loss. This seems like an enormous black hole in our knowledge because the previous and following scenarios happen way too often.

The husband is sixty. He wears expensive clothes that make him look hot, he has an impressive automobile, has achieved an obvious level of financial growth, and has pretty much kept his college weight (except for that little Buddha belly that somehow looks adorable on men). He is surviving in a sexless marriage to a woman who is struggling valiantly to get through each day with a little help from multiple pharmaceuticals that are not working to her benefit.

As carbon-based life forms of human protoplasm, humans have not yet evolved to be egoless. Most have evolved to be nice, but not to be kind. The husband is feeling neglected, unloved, and lonely. Men not only need sex, they need attention and affirmation of their daily warrior efforts. Home is not a happy place.

Not to worry. The husband happens upon a thirty-five or forty-something woman who thinks he is the best thing since the invention of the iPhone. She *smiles* when she sees him. They talk and open up to each other about their plans and dreams. They text and have an emotional twenty-first century e-mail affair. Then it happens. They accidentally touch. The electromagnetic force field can be registered on the Richter scale.

Time marches on. On the boardwalk, I pass this former husband of wife number one who lost one-half of his worldly goods and possibly the respect of his children. He is *pushing a baby carriage,* a state of the art model that does everything, even plays Baby Einstein DVDs.

The point here is, this man didn't want a baby, he wanted sex. He takes Viagra, which may not always work to his liking. He wanted companionship with the mother of his children, and affirmation of his journey. This is a sad story that did not have to happen. The American medical model failed.

But, out of bad can come good. All the *problems* were chaos to be welcomed. All the chaos had a solution, but as doctors trained in America, we didn't learn how to help this family. Unless your doctor studies a lot and goes to conferences with amazing endocrinologists from near and far, he/she may not have a solution for you, but one does exist.

Your Wife Wants Sex, Not a Baby

Young men about to start a family know their wives want that baby. Ask an older group of men married to women between the ages of forty and seventy if the title for this section makes any sense to them, and a significant number might say, "No, my wife doesn't want either." Obviously this is the group not having sex, who can't see the truth in this title. Change the word sex to *attention* and it will make much more sense to them.

People state that, especially after the childbearing years, they are no longer having sexual relations at home and they are frustrated. Their mates find one excuse or another to avoid sex. Sometimes, in the middle of an attempt, one or the other will bring up an issue that starts a fight, and it almost feels planned to avoid a sexual encounter. Eventually, many of the guys stop *begging* for sex, to use their words. Some move towards pornography, others venture out to the local strip clubs, and others actually find a new love interest, whether it's at work, online, or at a bar.

Men are wise to learn that women need sex too. For those women who seem disinterested in sex later in life, they need attention. With appropriate attention the sexual relationship can be revived. The sexual and affection needs of women are generally met in the early stages of marriage, as are those of men. The problem arises when men become so busy they forget that their wives are sexual creatures and need to be attended to, just like them.

Women may also find other sexual outlets when unattended to, such as becoming involved in an affair, or socializing with friends in places that may lead to sexual encounters. Even Internet encounters have become a way for some women to get the attention and sex they miss at home.

The critical mistake is that rather than trying to find a solution to their problem at home, many couples allow the marriage to fall apart. They are amazed to find out their seemingly asexual mate who had been rejecting their sexual attempts actually leaves them for another. "What was wrong? How did this person break through while I was rejected all those years?" Remember, you both need sexual fulfillment and attention.

Taboo and You

Although divorce was a well-respected taboo for most of American history, over the past forty-five years it has been pretty much eviscerated.[5] No longer does anyone have to live in a sexless marriage. No longer will anyone be judged for seeking a divorce.

Adultery

For most cultures, adultery has been a taboo since the beginning of history. In contemporary America it is no longer the bearer of the scarlet letter. While it may not be openly accepted, adultery is tolerated. Because it is no longer the effective taboo it once was, adultery is being used as a way to escape the sexless marriage, instead of the conventional methods of counseling, separation, and divorce.[6]

Pornography

Fifty years ago it was difficult to find, but today pornography is a multi-billion dollar industry—it is everywhere, including on most hotel-room television sets. Pornography is a double-edge sword for a relationship—in some cases, it is a lifesaver, but in other cases it keeps the relationship sexless. While it may relieve some of the frustration of a sexless marriage, it can also keep the sexually active partner so satisfied that he/she may not feel any reason to work on the fractured relationship.

Prostitution

Touted as the oldest profession, prostitution has been, and continues to be, illegal in most jurisdictions, making it risky and avoided by many. However, since the taboo and stigma associated with prostitution is dead, it has never been more available than it is today. Frustrated men who might never entertain an adulterous relationship are more than ever willing to use prostitution to revitalize their sexual prowess when it can no longer be satisfied in the marriage bed.

3

Understanding
the Forces of Attraction

Four Factors for Sex and Intimacy

BEING INTIMATE AND SEXUAL INVOLVES A COMBINATION OF EMO-
tional, hormonal, mental, and physical health. You may think of these
things as separate, but they all interact with one another. A successful
marriage is a symphony of players capable of maximizing these factors, with hormones playing an especially important role in how the
other three are affected.

You don't have to live life without sex. There are remedies for most
of the causes of sexless partnerships; however, you and your partner
have to *want* to fix the problems. What happens when your mate
doesn't think anything is wrong, or doesn't want to get help? If one of
you is depressed or has diminished hormones, you aren't very likely
to see the problem or have any interest in fixing it. If your partner
will not make any attempt to fix the problem, or your attempts fail,
there may come a time when you have to decide to either live under
these conditions or abandon the marriage vows and move on to a new
life. This is a personal issue, and only you can decide if your union
is *until death do you part.*

It would be ideal to have discussions about sex with your mate,
but quite often it remains a taboo subject, especially when things
aren't right. Getting help, or getting the right help, won't just happen.
You will have to make it happen. It begins with a conversation that
should be compassionate and may go like this: "Honey," (don't use

that name if you didn't before) "We need to talk. I feel our love life is suffering, and I would like to understand why and do something about it." Notice here the need to talk about your *feelings* and *understanding*. This is not the time to be accusatory or harsh.

You really have to be ready for anything. Wouldn't you want to know about a third person now, allowing you to realize your mate has a divided heart that requires attention, rather than leading a sexless life while he/she spreads his/her energy elsewhere? Hopefully, you have not pressed the cruise control button. Just like plants need sunshine, water, and attention, marital partners need tending as well. Most importantly, he/she needs to be heard, usually a hallmark of a *new relationship* (i.e. the affair). If neither of you is interested in the sexual component of your relationship, there's no problem. If one of you knows the other is getting attention elsewhere, and you don't care, no problem—until you get served with divorce papers. The real problem may be that one or the other is deceived into thinking their mate is sexless when they are not.

It is surprising how many men and women are shocked when their spouses leave them. Those to whom it should be no surprise are those who have been unhappy and sexless for years. Other men and women can actually believe their marital life is great and their spouse is happy. For them, it is either a misconception about how great their love life and compatibility really were, or their spouse may be going through a crisis of sorts—midlife now seems to extend to any age—or even having sexual preference issues.

Desire

Desire is a longing or craving for something that offers satisfaction or enjoyment. Many things can be desired. *Sex is a primal desire.* As much as we may like to think we are above such primitive longings because of our evolutionary development, we are not. Strides have been made to allow us to be societal in nature, and most people don't engage in sex with complete abandon. There are certain dictates that keep people out of harm's way and punish those who cannot contain themselves. However, the reality is that with all the taboos, restraints, prohibitions, and laws regarding sexuality, people are still very much influenced by the primal element of desire.

There is a reason a sixteen-year-old boy is capable of mating with anyone or anything, including inanimate objects, as so very vividly pictured in the movie *American Pie*. The reason is best described by an explosion of hormones, specifically, *testosterone* which is the hormone of sexual desire (libido).[1]

The same holds true for women, though to a lesser extent. As the female explodes with her hormonal cascade, she becomes interested in sexual activity. And while the woman is usually more discreet, there is still a strong desire to connect with another.

The decline of sexual desire is a major reason marriages become sexless. The complexity of this premise is due to the multitude of factors that cause this decline of desire. Some understanding of the causes of lost libido are needed in order to fix them.

Emotional Support

Emotional support or need may also play a significant role in desire. To some degree, loneliness is remedied, at least for the moment, by engaging in sexual activity, and for some, their desire is based on feeding this need.

Hormones

Hormones provide sexual desire (aka *libido*), but they also play a major role in mood, depression, and many aspects of physical health. Hormones work together and every hormone has hundreds of jobs to perform.

Cerebral Component and Chemistry

Hormones are not the only factor to influence desire. There is a cerebral component that stimulates desire. Sex starts in the brain. Sometimes it's called chemistry. It may be a certain facial characteristic, a body shape, intellectual prowess; the list is long. It includes anything imaginable that one person or another finds desirable.

Then there are the changes in looks, bodies, and interests that may have made two people so incompatible over the years that their mates may wonder what they ever found desirable. Just as looks and behavior can change over time, chemistry can fade. Many take it for granted that chemistry is forever—it isn't.

Therapy's Goal—To Rekindle Desire

The goal of therapy for the sexless marriage is to rekindle desire. This long-sought-after and ever-elusive aphrodisiac is really what it's all about. For some, pornography or sexy attire lights a fire; for others, flowers, a sentimental card, or a foot rub reignites the desire to bond sexually. A part of the brain called the hypothalamus stimulates desire, and hormones make it happen.

Libido—Deprivation—Satisfaction—Satiation

Like most things in life, there are different levels of libido for different people. Libido varies at different times of the day, week, month, and life cycle. It is also held to the whim of a feedback mechanism[2] where *the more you get, the less you want, and the less you get, the more you want*—that is, assuming all other systems are in order and you haven't been deprived for too long. This is why men very often want to turn over and go to sleep after sexual climax. Their libido has been satisfied and it's time to say goodnight. Sure, there are biological reasons for this fulfillment, but the result is satisfaction. If they are the type who wishes to go for a second and third round, satisfaction may be difficult to come by, and that type of individual may be difficult to please. There are some people who have libidinal needs beyond what is deemed typical. If they don't find a mate who can keep up, they may be on the prowl. Hopefully, you will find out if your libidos are reasonably compatible before you make marital commitments.

From a sexual perspective, the key for men and women who want to keep their partners from straying involves learning to keep them from experiencing libido deprivation—make sure they exist in mostly libido satisfaction and back off when they are in a state of libido satiation. The hard part is to know when each stage is broached and act accordingly. The only way to do this right is to learn to read your mate and make sure you can communicate with one another. This communication requires both parties to be heard, feel safe, and trust one another.

Relationships

The subject of this book is not limited to *marital* relationships. Many people in meaningful relationships are not married. Whatever the relationship is called: "My S.O. (significant other), my lady/guy friend," . . . and in Europe, "my lover," marital and monogamous relationships come with the assumption that the couple is, or was at some time, sexual.

Some marriages have slowly evolved into being roommates. The reality of what is happening behind closed doors is disquieting. Husbands and wives are saying to each other, "I don't want a roommate. I want my husband/wife back. What happened to the person I married?"

Is there an alternative to a sexless marriage? Withdrawing from intimate communion is an alternative, but it doesn't work if both partners are not on board. My experience with patients is that the loss of sex in their relationships leads to repressed anger, confusion, feelings of rejection, new-onset addictions, such as overeating, over-exercising, over-thinking, over-shopping . . . the list continues. The very force that brought many folks together fades away, leading to loneliness. Dating couples may easily walk away from sexless relationships. Married couples, however, must go through a lengthy legal process that usually results in a physical, emotional, financial, and spiritually agonizing experience. Divorce is a death without a death.

There are many forces that lead to the demise of sex in relationships. By understanding these forces, you can learn, in every possible way, to rebuild the strong bond with the person you once loved.

There are many sexless couples who reason that they now have, "something better, something deeper, a relationship in which sex is no longer important." Try telling a sexually active couple that one day they will have a better relationship once the sex is gone. Their response will be, "Yeah, right."

In our opinion (RF, RM), the only time the loss of sexuality is acceptable is when one or both mates are physically unable to be sexually intimate. Later, you will learn that there are medical remedies for many conditions that lead couples to think they have forever lost the ability to be sexual.

Whether you are in a marriage, dating, or have a friend-with-benefits relationship, it takes much effort to keep it alive. Make your brain indelibly aware of the phrase, *it takes work to make the relationship work.*

But what does that actually mean?

Some of the reasons relationships don't work are: being too busy with work, family, and individual interests to engage as you once did; being too content with daily life; adopting complacency in your appearance; no longer bringing life to the union with learning; trying new things . . . all those put a crimp in relationships.

The most overpowering alternative is the replacement of lost love with another beloved. This new beloved listens to your hopes, dreams, and concerns. They *really* listen. For some, being heard is more important than being loved—actually, being heard is being loved.

The Role of Sex in Relationships

How important is sex in a relationship? There are several ways to quantify this answer.

The Time Perspective

From a time perspective, a normal relationship finds couples engaging in sex for around ten minutes to four hours a week (age- and libido-dependent). So, on a time basis, sex, on average, occupies less than one-percent of your life—most folks spend more time waiting at red lights than having sex.

You need to ask yourself how something that takes up so little time in relationships can be so very important? How come there never seems to be the time to engage in this activity that takes up so little time? It must be because time in minutes and hours isn't everything when it comes to sex.

Frequency

Frequency of sexual activity is a big factor in relationship satisfaction. If you find yourself not having sex frequently enough, then it matters 99 percent.

Conversely, if there is too much sex for one of the partners, they, too, find sex to be 99 percent important in their relationship. Too much, just like too little sex in your life, both result in frustration, anger, resentment, and discontentment.

Before You Get Married—Again

There are several important things to keep in mind when contemplating a remarriage.

Compatibility

When getting into a meaningful relationship, the first thing to consider is compatibility. This is true whether it's your first marriage or a subsequent one. It may seem obvious, but it's surprising how many people don't give compatibility much thought. Oftentimes, especially with younger couples, relationships are based on what is commonly thought of as lust. If lust is the foundation of a relationship, then when it fades, which nature seems to consider inevitable, the couple finds themselves with little reason to remain together.

Common Interests

Along with general compatibility, and of course, sexual compatibility, common interests must be considered before you marry. Do the two of you have things to do *together*? Are your separate interests (also necessary) so time-consuming that you will neglect your partner, or does your partner, too, have a busy enough schedule or interests to keep occupied? Common interests allow for a relationship that is broad-based and not grounded in sex alone.

The Goldilocks Rule of Sex

Another important consideration could be called *The Goldilocks Rule*—not too much and not too little sex. This needs to come into play because sexual frequency and quality has to be just right. Ask, or try to figure out, exactly how much sex this person desires to remain in a committed relationship. A good test to check for this requires some simple questions that, if answered truthfully, will allow you to start out on the right track.

At some point in the courting stage, ask your mate how often it would be good to engage in sex on a weekly basis. This should be stated as a multiple choice question: once a week, at least once a week, one or two times a week, *at least* one or two times a week, two or three times a week, *at least* two or three times a week, and so on. Notice there is a distinction drawn here between wanting to have sex a certain number of times a week and *at least* a certain number of times a week. *At least* is a very important qualifier, because when a mate says they want to engage in sex two or three times a week, they may be suggesting what they think they want, with some reservation, or they may be saying what they think *you* want.

The Honeymoon Phase

In the early stages of relationships, things are usually at their best. Everyone is on their best behavior, the sex is good, and you are in the honeymoon phase. Sex may be so good that it clouds your thinking, allowing you to forget all the other components of a good relationship. As you've no doubt heard, however, honeymoons don't last forever, at least not without much hard work. And that includes finding out upfront what your common interests are, and what incompatibilities you may have. If you ignore or gloss over these aspects of each other, then you're setting your relationship up for disaster.

Treatment Options

Six Reasons for Sexual Decline and Six Primary Treatments

1. Behavioral issues

2. Financial issues

3. Hormonal issues

4. Personal issues

5. Physical and health-related issues

6. Psychological issues

Any of the above, or a combination of two or more of them may be the primary reasons for diminished sexual activity.

There are also six primary treatments to manage these problems. They are:

1. Behavior modification

2. Managing general health issues

3. Hormonal therapy

4. Lifestyle changes, including financial adjustments

5. Natural supplements and prescription medications

6. Psychotherapy

After a brief look at each treatment, they will be applied to the dysfunction to which they could relate.

Behavior Modification

Also known as attitude adjustment, behavior modification is required to manage the many personal and behavioral issues described in that chapter. You will never achieve a healthy sexual relationship if you continue to treat your mate poorly.

General Health Issues

General health issues could be the source of your sexless marriage. They need to be explored. Diabetes, heart disease, obesity, and spinal injuries are only a few of the ailments that can affect sexual relationships. Doctor-guided blood-sugar control, cardiac care, diet treatment, and pain-control remedies can get you back into the game. Gynecological and urological problems must be addressed to make sex happen if those systems fail you.

Hormonal Issues

With regard to the hormonal issues that are such a strong component of the sexless marriage, your doctor may decide to prescribe replacement hormones. These hormones can make a big difference in helping to solve many of the symptoms related to sexless relationships. If hormones are needed, however, make sure you find a doctor who can guide you in the use of bio-identical hormones.

Lifestyle Changes

It is always preferable to solve health-related and personal problems with lifestyle changes. Eliminating destructive behaviors and making healthy choices are the safest and best long-term solutions. It is common knowledge that eating a healthy diet high in fruits and vegetables and low in sugar and saturated fat, maintaining a healthy body weight, not smoking, getting plenty of sleep, and regular exercise, have huge payoffs in terms of how you feel and function—especially sexually. Unfortunately, for many, these things are too difficult. Results may not be immediately apparent, but the value to the quality of life cannot be overestimated. There are many programs available to help a person quit smoking or lose weight, but starting and sticking with whichever one you choose is key. It is easy to pop a pill in a society that is always searching for the easy fix, but pills alone will not be as effective as a combined approach with a healthy lifestyle.

Natural Supplementation

Supplementation ranges from vitamin and mineral replacement to herbal or homeopathic remedies. Many are effective, though some might not do anything particular for you. If you plan on self-medicating, you have to do your homework or find a trusted healer to guide you on the selection of effective, safe remedies. Whatever forms of treatments you and your doctor consider, make sure to indicate your interest in using natural remedies and products rather than jumping to the prescription medications.

Prescription Drugs

Although prescription drugs may not be the best way to go, they are often easiest way. Even though they are heavily tested for toxicity and are monitored by a doctor, many prove to be dangerous, even after FDA approval. And of course, every drug does not work for every person with similar symptoms—there is no *one size fits all* with drugs. Trial and error may be required. This is especially true with antidepressants that, in addition, may take up to four weeks to begin to work. The advantage of prescription therapy is that when you and your doctor find the right treatment, it can be like the sun coming out after a storm. Drugs may help relieve depression, enhance libido, and treat erectile dysfunction, all helping to remedy the sexless marriage.

Psychological Issues

Psychological problems leading to a sexless marriage can be related to life situations, chemical imbalances of brain chemicals, or hormone imbalances that affect brain chemicals. These problems could develop from many sources—the trauma of rape, incest, or post-traumatic stress disorder (PTSD) from any cause—alcoholism, depression related to chemical imbalances in the brain, or sadness from some type of loss. While talk therapy (psychotherapy) may help in getting to the source of a problem and in dealing with life issues, it is not always enough. Prescription medication may sometimes be needed to manage imbalances, but be aware of medication's catch-22 for depression—some drugs cause sexual dysfunction or loss of libido. If you do choose to use medications, don't wait too long to begin the appropriate ones.

All About Women— Female Sexuality

SEX IS THE EMOTIONAL HUMAN CRAZY GLUE THAT INADVERTENTLY made you believe that you and your partner in sex were a couple, and sex will help you transform those occasions when you look at the other one in the relationship and wonder, "What the hell happened? We were so close." That time arrives when the relationship stumbles and one or both of you needs an injection of reality so you can grow up. In most failed marriages, whatever the stumbling block is, it will be moved to the new, perfect relationship you went on to form. Perhaps learning about your sexuality in the current relationship will help it stay intact.

How well do you understand your mate's sexuality? Little boys are fascinated with their penises. They look at them and touch them. Onlookers think it's cute or tell them to do that only when alone. They are given room to experiment, and it feels normal. Little girls are told to *stop that*. They are made to feel dirty or abnormal and there's no room given them to experiment. Little girls wear white dresses for special occasions and these are intended to signify their purity. A lot of women reach adulthood without having any idea what an orgasm feels like. Societal dictates, mores, and values do affect male and female sexuality differently.

Some Facts You Should Know about Female Sexuality

As a rule, women don't look at their genitalia. Ask a woman if she knows where her clitoris is (an inch or two above the vaginal opening), or where her G-spot is (approximately an inch and a half inside the vagina on the front side of the vaginal canal), and many won't know. Women need to know where their clitoris and G-spot are located. They need to be encouraged to experiment, play, and have fun with sex and sexuality.

Sex begins in the brain. The hypothalamus in the brain is a powerful aphrodisiac. Want to spark her desire? Take the trash out. Listen to what she says. Be really nice to her even when she is not naked.

An orgasm causes the levels of oxytocin to increase five to ten fold in both men and women. Why oxytocin, the hormone that allows the uterus to contract during childbirth?[1] High levels of oxytocin create attachment between partners. European endocrinologists have explained that oxytocin also enhances a couple's feeling of closeness and tenderness with each other. If it sounds good so far, there's more. Oxytocin makes all the other brain neurotransmitters work better.[2] Oh, and women need testosterone as well. They make 1/10 the amount of testosterone as men, and it declines after menopause. Since testosterone is a big part of both the decline of desire for sex and the decline of muscle mass and skin tone, I (RM) prescribe low-dose pharmaceutically compounded testosterone gel. My patients tell me that first they have a sexual dream. Then, when their husbands want to have relations, they find themselves receptive. They may even begin to initiate. They don't say, "Oh darn."

Some women do well with transdermal cream, some do well with transdermal gel, some do well with testosterone taken by injection, and some require the vaginal formulation containing more than just testosterone. You and your doctor may have to experiment to find what works best.

So, testosterone isn't just for men anymore. And sex isn't just for men any more. Welcome to the millennium.

Can Women Achieve Orgasm
Via Penile Penetration Alone?

Sigmund Freud described female sexuality as a dark continent[3] and described two types of orgasm: clitoral orgasm from masturbation (which Freud said was immature) and vaginal orgasm via intercourse (which Freud said was the mature kind).4 Apparently, there was a right and wrong way to do it. And so began the confusion: Is something wrong with women who cannot achieve penis-in-vagina orgasm?

Most women who cannot experience orgasm via penile penetration alone feel inadequate. They feel guilty when they need clitoral stimulation to achieve orgasm, or they fake an orgasm because they don't want their husbands to feel inadequate. Then they feel inadequate instead because they have not communicated what they need to have an orgasm.

The first person to say what determines whether or not a woman can achieve orgasm by intercourse alone was Marie Bonaparte, a twentieth-century French aristocrat and a great-grand niece to Napoleon. Marie was a very sensual, but very frustrated woman because she couldn't achieve orgasm during sexual intercourse with her husband. After many unsuccessful consultations with renowned physicians, she came up with a theory after she discovered there was a wide span between her clitoris and her vagina.

Following up on her theory, Marie assembled a group of 243 women and measured the distance between the two body parts, then asked each woman how easily she could achieve orgasm via intercourse. She found a correlation. If the distance was greater than one and a half inches, vaginal orgasm was not possible.5 Who knew? Female genitalia anatomy is quite complex. Without a mirror and a pictorial of your womanliness to serve as your tour guide, would you know what your minor and major vulva or clitoral glans and clitoral hood look like? Would you even think that the length between your vaginal introitus (opening) and clitoral hood is advantageously short, too long, or just right?

Eventually science caught up with Marie Bonaparte. Biology professor Elisabeth Lloyd at Indiana University turned Bonaparte's anecdotally proven theory into a scientific study. The results were fascinating. Lloyd discovered that if the distance between the vaginal opening and clitoral hood is longer than the distance between the tip of the thumb and the first knuckle, women were unable to achieve orgasm with penile penetration alone. Lloyd called this *the rule of thumb*.6 There are as many statistics out there as there are studies. Due to many variables in the design of the studies and those who participate, you can quote a wide range of numbers concerning women and orgasm. To simplify this, a quote from a recent report stated that around 75 percent of women are unable to reach orgasm from intercourse alone (*ABC News*, September 4, 2009). With the help of sex toys, hands, or tongue providing clitoral stimulation, that number drops to around 10–15 percent.

The Clitoral Orgasm

In the 1950s, Alfred Kinsey released *Sexual Behavior in the Human Female*. Everything changed. Kinsey concluded that the clitoris, not the vagina, was the central pleasure receptor for women.[7] In their 1966 book, *Human Sexual Response*, researchers Masters and Johnson posited that the clitoris extended beyond the clitoral glans and shaft to include several areas behind the labia. They concluded that all orgasms, even those that occurred through intercourse alone, were therefore clitoral orgasms.[8]

Why Do Women Fake Orgasms?

University of Indiana researchers conducted the National Survey of Sexual Health and Behavior and found that 85 percent of men thought women reached orgasm, while actually, only 64 percent of women agreed. This came to be called the orgasm gap. Apparently the fact that women can fake it and men can't tell that they have holds true even in scientific study. Apparently having an orgasm is still a concern for many women.[9]

Women know there is a lot of pressure on men to please them. They want their husbands to think they have made them happy. By faking orgasms, women achieve this goal with the result that they may be missing out on the full pleasure of sexual union.

The G-Spot

In 1950, a German gynecologist, Ernest Gräfenberg, identified several erogenous zones located on the front wall of the vagina. He published a paper about sexual satisfaction and orgasm in women entitled, *The*

Role of Urethra in Female Orgasm, in which he identified a sensitive area inside and to the front of the vagina, near the pubic bone. The claim was that the urethra is surrounded by erectile tissue that swells during stimulation and that some women *expel fluid* from the urethra at the moment of orgasm, and the fluid is not urine, it is female ejaculation.[10]

The area described by Dr. Ernst Gräfenberg in his research was what later came to be called the "G-spot." The G-spot was described by Masters and Johnson to feel like a small bean, and, when a woman was aroused, it could swell to the size of a half-dollar. They suggested that if a woman was not aroused, it was because the G-spot was difficult, if not impossible, to find.

Debates continue within academic and scientific communities about the existence of the G-spot and its role in female pleasure. There is no need to debate in the bedroom. You and your partner should explore what feels good. Don't be afraid to show and tell your partner how to enhance your pleasure. Change positions, try sex toys, extend foreplay, until you find what works best.

Female Ejaculation

Female ejaculation is a much researched and debated topic. Many believe the female ejaculate is urine, but tests have proved it is actually fluid produced by women's skene glands near the urethra.

Most women contract their vaginal vault and uterus inward when they climax. Women who ejaculate report they push outwards when they climax, like they are going to urinate.

Female ejaculators report that their orgasms are so strong they feel very intense pleasure. If there is a controversy over whether female ejaculation really exists, why has it been described in several ancient texts, including the *Kama Sutra,* the more than 2,000-year-old revered treatise on sexuality? Most women can learn to ejaculate if they so desire and have a patient husband who wants to please his wife in a new way.

Menopause and Sex

Women have a well-known name for their age-related plight. It's called menopause. Most everyone has heard of menopause. While their understanding may be limited, the big picture is that most women have hot flashes, become moody, and may lose interest in sex. Upon further study, however, it's apparent that menopause is much more complicated than just three symptoms.

In addition to what are so prevalently presented as the cardinal menopausal symptoms, namely hot flashes and vaginal dryness, women tell me they can no longer sleep, think, remember, keep their moods in check, conjure any interest in being sexual, or maintain their weight. Add to this scenario palpitations, loss of bone, occasionally debilitating depression, with loss of motivation and focus and changes in skin. The menopausal woman's complaint is usually more than one thing, and the chief one is, "Doctor, my life has been taken away. Please listen to me and help me!" Sadly, however, the doctor will often skim over this blanket statement because it does not fit well with the current medical model where you give your doctor a complaint and in return you will be given one prescription to take care of the issue.

For the first forty to fifty years of life, women are making hormones in their ovaries, adrenal glands, skin, brain, and thyroid, then they begin to have a decline. When you put the hormonal deficiency in the blender with the person's history of overwork, unrelenting stressors, and their overeating of nutrient-deficient, rich foods, you have a recipe for the disaster that has manifested in earnest and has resulted in a sexless marriage, with the potential to see the dissolution of the entire marriage if it is not properly fixed.

It's Not Just About Menopause

Today not being in the mood is more often called hypoactive sexual desire disorder than frigidity. Then there is vaginismus. Though rare, this is a condition where the vagina closes down and becomes impenetrable. Other problems that may have negative effects on a woman's libido include the effects of a hysterectomy, hormonal imbalances that can occur at any age, not just in menopause, valvodynia (sensitivity around the vagina), dyspenunia (pain inside the vagina), orgasmic disorder, sexual abuse, post-traumatic syndrome, certain medications (antidepressants and anti-anxiety drugs), drug and/or alcohol abuse, smoking, and stress.

Premenstrual Syndrome—PMS

The most common hormonal issue seen in young women is premenstrual syndrome (PMS). When assessing the mental state of women, questions regarding depression, moodiness, feelings of loneliness, temper, and frustration all come into play. It's not that men don't have many of the same issues, but, generally speaking, PMS symptoms in a young woman can recur monthly and are not easily treated with antidepressants alone.

PMS is the cause of many sexless relationships, and much frustration and angst for both the women experiencing the symptoms and the men who have to cope with them. Marriages can fail under the strain.

Solutions for Women's Issues

Depression, Anxiety, and Other Psychological Problems

Unfortunately, many practitioners (often family practice physicians or gynecologists) treat depression and anxiety by prescribing the quick-fix antidepressants, with no recommendation for counseling. This type of limited care may help symptoms, but without addressing the underlying causes, the chances of getting well and improving interpersonal relationships are poor.

Once all physical and hormonal problems that can cause psychological troubles are ruled out or addressed, it might become necessary to get care from either a psychologist (who uses talk therapy), a psychiatrist (who usually prescribes medications), or, more likely, both.

Libido and orgasm issues unrelated to hormones, physical, and/or depressive illness may require treatment by a certified sex therapist—they do exist. You might consider games to play with your mate, sex toys, sexually explicit books, or movies. It is not the scope of this book to treat the many psychological issues that can result in the sexless marriage, but rather to point you toward the appropriate care.

Irreconcilable Differences

There must be the realization that some people, women and men alike, are asexual and very much content. To try and make a zebra into a horse will fail. In the course of human relationships, there may come a time when you must recognize an incompatibility that offers nothing but frustration to both parties. In situations like this, *irreconcilable* ones in the divorce-court jargon, you have to decide between living in frustration, living in an open marriage, or getting a separation or a divorce. None of these remedies are without problems of their own. You should do some soul-searching before you take the leap. If you have tried all the available therapies and remedies, at least you will know you have made a good effort if you do decide to separate.

Hormonal Problems

The possibility of hormone imbalances requires evaluation and treatment by a medical doctor experienced in this area. It is imperative to find a practitioner well-versed in hormonal issues—specifically bio-identical hormones—as required in the treatment of menopause or PMS. Unless your doctor (gynecologist, endocrinologist, internist, etc) has good knowledge of all aspects of hormonal treatment, he/she may either make light of, or ignore, the problems. Let the knowledge you have gained here direct you to pursue a good doctor with the proper training and expertise to help you or your loved one.

MEDICATION MISTAKE

Laura K, a sixty-year-old woman with a history of ovary removal, came to see me (RM). She was beginning to lose her hair and was having difficulty achieving orgasm even though she thoroughly enjoyed engaging in sex frequently. Her gynecologist had prescribed the drug Activella, a combination pill containing estradiol and norethindrone (a progestin-synthetic progesterone).

While this medication is prescribed by many doctors, it is not a good choice in my opinion. Take a look at the warning on this medication. It flat out tells you that postmenopausal women taking estrogen with progestins, exactly what is found in Activella, can increase their risk of heart attack, stroke, lung clots, breast cancer, ovarian cysts and other problems.[11] As mentioned numerous times in this book, it is the progestin (synthetic progesterone) that is the danger, not the estrogen or natural progesterone.

When asked if there were any recent changes in her blood levels of the associated hormones she had been prescribed, Laura said she would have to call her doctor to find out. At a subsequent visit, she said she found out that her gynecologist had never ordered any blood tests to determine her hormone levels.

This manner of treatment happens all too often. How can a medical professional prescribe potent hormones for many years, and in this case, synthetic hormones known to have many associated risks, and never check the level of hormones? This is not good practice. Yet these very same doctors criticize bio-identical hormone replacement because they truly don't understand what it is all about.

Even though Activella has a natural estrogen, it is not safe. Taking estrogen in pill form allows it to concentrate in the liver and increase SHBG (sex hormone-binding globulin that ties up your hormones). Its side effects include depression, mood changes, confusion, memory loss, breast lumps, unusual vaginal bleeding, and more.[12]

Blood tests and appropriate bio-identical hormone replacement were prescribed for Laura, and within two months her hair was no longer falling out and had returned to its fullness. Her levels of progesterone and estrogen were brought back to youthful levels, as shown by her continued blood testing.

Proper hormone levels should serve her well in maintaining good health. Orgasms for her remained unpredictable—bio-identical hormone replacement therapy (BHRT) is not always a cure-all. People need to recognize that just because there is one positive result of so many possible causes to the various problems, there may not be just one solution.

In 1995, Dr. Morgan, this book's co-author, was the Medical Director of the internationally acclaimed Princeton Bio Center—according to her, a stroke of luck on her part. During that time, a schizophrenic woman told her she was unable to reach orgasm when she took her medication. And, when she didn't reach orgasm, the voices (her hallucinations) got more intense and frequent. This woman was saying that sexuality is not only important for procreation and recreation, but also for mental health—women, you need sex.

Between 70–80 percent of women never have a penis-in-vagina orgasm.[13] As in *Seinfeld* episodes and *When Harry Met Sally*, they are faking. Unless the architecture between a man and a woman is compatible, or they experiment with sexual positions that allow for more clitoral/ penile contact, most women are unable to have a penis-in-vagina orgasm. They find, instead, that independent clitoral stimulation is more likely to result in orgasm. Some women have a hooded clitoris, making stimulation difficult. Some women require thyroid hormone, as thyroid increases the blood flow to the clitoris, the vulva, and the entire area. This is analogous to a man's erection—increased blood flow to the penis (a very simplified description), which is how Viagra works. Viagra works for some of my women patients as well, and my speculation is that it most probably will receive FDA approval for use with women in the future, even though, current research doesn't support this view.

Maximizing Female Orgasms

The University of Indiana National Survey of Sexual Health and Behavior study, noted above, showed that there are ways to maximize achieving an orgasm. While vaginal intercourse was still the most common sexual behavior, they found that men and women rarely engage in just one type of sex. They found that women who engage in a greater number and variety of sexual encounters during their most recent partnered sex acts are more likely to report having an orgasm.

Perhaps by adding some variety to your sexual repertoire, you will improve your sexual experience. Different positions, oral sex, masturbation, and pornographic movies all offer enhanced sexuality and may help restore some excitement to the bedroom, and, as such, should be considered. Vibrators and other sex toys are a great shortcut to orgasms. Finding out what works best and what you are capable of in the pleasure department is a boon for any woman of any age. There are weekend conferences where women can learn about their sexuality, examine themselves for the first time, and learn to masturbate to orgasm—truly.

There are many good, free, resources online for learning new sexual positions. Consider romantic novels to add excitement to your life. An empire of instructional sexual videos is available to enhance what is happening in your bedroom. Kathy Brummitt, the director of production at BetterSex.com, has been teaching couples how to make love for decades. The Sinclair Institute produces and markets adult sex-education videos with over seventy titles on subjects from how to become orgasmic, for women, to premature ejaculation, for males, bondage videos, anal sex videos, female ejaculation, and the list goes on. Sex should be fun.

Why is there increased variety in sexual behavior today compared to 1950? Simple. There was no birth control pill in 1950. The pill allowed sex to transform from procreation only to procreation and recreation. The book, *The Joy of Sex*, first published in 1972, was frank and candid and lit a fire under our anemic sexual proclivities. The book has been updated for the twenty-first century.[14]

Even in marriage, men are big fans of masturbation. Women masturbate too, sometimes when they are angry or frustrated with men. Actually, occasional masturbation is normal in a marriage, but it should not be the prime source of sexual gratification unless your sexual needs are not in sync, or if you are in a consensual sexless marriage.

Sex shapes people and potentiates the ability to love, enjoy life, and each other. But for sex to happen, you have to feel safe. You have to feel accepted. You have to be heard. You have to be able to trust the other before merging. Then you can connect emotionally, and sex is the joyous result of the trust and connection. It is just like the intimate communion that made you think it was time to stop dating and get married.

Learn How To Be a Good—strike that—Great Lover

Now that many of your womanly issues have been covered, it's time to bring it all together. Your performance in the bedroom is just as important as his. Quite often the things you and your husband like are different. There are some things you should do, as well as some things you should not do.

For some odd reason, women (and some men) can bring up topics of daily interest in the middle of foreplay. This is nearly always not the time to discuss anything unrelated to your sexual bonding. Sex requires stimulation of the brain. When secular, everyday activities are discussed, the sex center of the brain gets sidetracked and ultimately turned off.

To make matters worse, if your man is working his way through erectile dysfunction issues, his erection will likely fade the moment you ask about getting an appointment to have the car serviced. Not the time for that conversation.

Anticipation is a great sex tool. You probably don't like your man to go right for your clitoris and prefer that he goes slowly. To the contrary, though, he does want you to go right to his penis, but take note that teasing can build tremendous sexual energy. Rub, massage, and feather-touch his neck, shoulders, chest, and stomach, all while working towards the end point. Move closer to the target and then back away. Move closer and then retreat. Make sure he never knows when you will actually move on to ground zero. There is no need to rush the process. Wouldn't it be nice if sexual activities could last longer? Try to avoid engaging in predictable sexual behaviors. The whole point is excited anticipation. Even though guys like to get right to work, the anticipation that comes from this type of foreplay puts you in the category of being a great lover.

Your guy usually likes to be stimulated by many senses. Wear a nice perfume that he often compliments, play some likeable music for the event, make sounds of ecstasy to let him know he's pleasing you and to enhance his desire. Breathe heavy even if you don't feel it because it gets him excited.

Oral sex (known as fellatio when performed on a man versus cunnilingus when performed on a woman) is highly exciting for those who engage in such activities. It adds to the repertoire of sexual engagement and allows for all sorts of anticipatory sensual moments. There are some women who are repulsed by the thought of engaging in oral sex and that issue may not be easily resolved. If, however, you want to please your man in a different manner, oral sex is something to consider. There are men who seek out other lovers to satisfy their quest for oral sex when their partners are not interested.

It is important to realize that many men are quickly excitable and anything the slightest bit kinky can set them off, so be careful that you don't overstimulate or the result may be premature ejaculation. Some guys are very sensitive about this. If he pulls your hand away, he is telling you to take it easy or he'll explode and he wants it to last longer. Men truly believe that if they don't last long, they are not good lovers (some women feel the same way). They want to please and they think the length of the lovemaking session and the length of the penis is what it's all about. Compliment your guy's prowess in bed and the size of his penis and he'll love you forever.

Once your man has entered the point of no return (called ejaculatory inevitability) he usually likes fast and firm stimulation. Regardless of whether it's actual penetration or stimulation by hand or mouth, go with the flow and follow his lead. Generally speaking, you don't want to ease up, slow down, or stop the motion during ejaculation. It can ruin the orgasm. Once he ejaculates, you will want to slow the pace, but keep some activity going as this helps expel all the ejaculate and gives him a feeling of satisfaction. In cases where he becomes hypersensitive (usually once the orgasm is completed), he will stop any motion and pull you away if necessary.

The male sex brain is exquisitely attuned to sexual activity. Young men think about sex often and are easily stimulated. Unless there is a testosterone deficiency, even older men think about sex a lot. It doesn't take much to excite most men. If you brush your breasts up against a guy's arm, he gets sexual thoughts, thinks you want him, and may even get an erection. If a guy brushes up against your breasts, you either don't even notice or just think he's clumsy. That sums up the differences between the male and female sex brain. A smart woman learns to use the guy's vulnerability to sexual stimuli to get him excited.

Remember when you first loved one another? There was pristine grooming, listening to each other, asking questions, doing things together, being affectionate and open to trying new activities and listening to new ideas. Sex was exploratory—you couldn't touch each other enough because you really liked one another and wanted to please. Although it's often said that sex will never be the same as those first early days, with knowledge and curiosity, it can actually be better. It's just that you already know what each other looks like in their birthday suit.

6

Women and Their Hormones

Progesterone

THERE ARE THINGS BOTH WOMEN AND MEN SHOULD UNDERSTAND about women and progesterone, and how it may affect relationships. If you are premenopausal and experiencing irregular periods, worsening premenstrual pain and menstrual cramps, heavier periods, missed periods, water retention, disabling anxiety, and very poor or no sleep, you aren't going to feel very sexual. It may be a good idea to check progesterone levels on approximately day twenty-one of your cycle (day one is the first day of menses). Many of these symptoms can be alleviated with an individualized dose of bio-identical progesterone cream or capsules. When you feel better, you may both feel better.

With supplementation of estrogen and progesterone, there is usually a fear of developing breast cancer. Balanced levels of bio-identical progesterone (*not* synthetic) protect against breast cancer. Technically, it does this by increasing P53, a substance that blocks BCL-2, which increases cancer. Progesterone also blocks COX-2, the urokinase plasminogen activator, and the nuclear factor-kappa beta (NFkB), which increases inflammation and the growth of cancer. Progesterone also protects breast tissue in women who have the HER-2/new oncogene, an aggressive breast-cancer marker which is present in 30 percent of women with breast cancer. In a French study on 54,000 women, those who used bio-identical progesterone had a 10-percent decrease in breast cancer.[1]

Bio-identical progesterone is good for you.

What we in the marine-corps-style—don't-ask-questions medical residency programs—are trained to prescribe is *synthetic progestin*. We are told it is the same as real progesterone. This is simply not true. Synthetic progestins are the reason the WHIS (Women's Health Initiative Study—see below) proved that hormone replacement therapy causes cancer.

The pharmaceutical companies quickly attempted to rescue the situation by developing a progesterone gel cap that is real progesterone, not synthetic progestin. This was a stellar move befitting the enormously powerful pharmaceutical companies. However, there are still a few drawbacks with the pharmaceutical progesterone known as Prometrium.

The Importance of Progesterone

Many women with the aforementioned laundry list of complaints get a prescription for a birth control pill. This is not for birth control. Rather, it is to curtail a growing list of symptoms. Some of these symptoms may come about because the pill eliminates all of a woman's natural progesterone production, which can cause a reduced libido, weight gain, inability to reach an orgasm, and an abnormal thyroid.

First, it behooves you to understand a bit about what progesterone does to make a woman a woman. It balances your estrogen so you have energy, a positive mood, and remain soft and calm.

(RM) Men tell me that their wives have become moody, labile, anxious, and depressed. They say, "This is not the woman I married." And women acknowledge that their husbands are telling the truth. But what is a woman to do? Should she take a tranquilizer that will dial the whole world down, causing her to live in a quasi-conscious state? That's not the answer.

The problem is most likely a lack of progesterone, which (especially in capsule form made by a compounding pharmacist) increases production of GABA (gamma amino butyric acid) and helps you remain calm and able to sleep. Pharmaceutical tranquilizers also contain GABA, but why take a tranquilizer that dulls everything when the GABA benefit can be gained with progesterone?

Most women work outside the home; they care for children, as well as parents who are not aging so well; they clean, cook, and don't sleep. Now a woman has a decision to make. Should she choose sleep or sex, sleep or sex, sleep or sex? She usually chooses sleep and prays that she can.

Progesterone works as a diuretic by decreasing another hormone called aldosterone (increased aldosterone increases water retention). Did you know that many women who commit murderous acts do so when they are just about to get their period?[2] The scientific reason for this (not the intellectual, spiritual, or emotional reason) is that their brains are retaining fluid that is pressing on areas of the brain that cause aggression. Progesterone comes to the rescue as it acts like a diuretic and decreases edema, or brain swelling. If progesterone could be properly balanced, then maybe those monthly psycho-unit, lockdown episodes could disappear and no longer be a new-onset dysfunctional ritual in your marriage.[3]

There are several reasons why the pharmaceutical-capsule variety of natural progesterone is inferior to the customized-dose type made by a compounding pharmacist.

1. First, the pharmaceutical form is suspended in peanut oil, a known allergen that can cause severe reactions in sensitive individuals.

2. Second, this gel cap available at your local pharmacy comes in only two doses: 100 and 200 mg. Women don't come in two sizes, so they respond differently to a one-dose-only prescription. The right dosage for you may be as low as 10 mg daily or as high as 500 mg daily, and it isn't easy to transform a 100 or 200 mg gel cap into an individually compounded dose.

Women require progesterone twenty-four hours a day. Progesterone taken by mouth peaks in blood levels within two to four hours and lasts for ten to fourteen hours. The nighttime dose of 100 mg is usually good for sleep, but most women report that the morning dose makes them feel sleepy. This is why a better alternative is a lower dose of transdermal progesterone in the morning, with an individualized, low-dose, micronized progesterone capsule made by a compounding pharmacist taken at bedtime. The dose gets adjusted until the woman can fall asleep and stay asleep. (If a woman experiences dizziness upon awakening, the dose is too high and needs adjusting.) This is how to restore progesterone in women so they can sleep and hopefully restore their libido.

Conventionally, doctors in the U.S. are trained that if a woman does not have a uterus, she doesn't require progesterone. This is *not true*. There are progesterone receptors from the top of your head to the tip of your toes. Women are often stressed out because they have so much to do that it is impossible to get everything done—even if they never slept. Progesterone is very calming. To get your calm back, you need *real* progesterone.

Natural progesterone cream is available over the counter in health food stores. The amount of actual progesterone may be too low to alleviate symptoms, but you can try it first to see if it helps. When it comes to hormones that should be monitored by regular blood tests, however, women need a licensed medical physician to prescribe the pharmaceutically compounded progesterone. This is a better alternative approach than the one-size-fits-all hormones made by the pharmaceutical companies. Each woman is unique, and requires a unique dose. The ideal dose of any hormone is extremely individualized and needs to be determined by ongoing blood tests to make sure a proper balance is maintained.

The WHIS Study

As a result of the July 2nd, 2002 conclusions regarding the Women's Health Initiative Study (WHIS), doctors, women, and the media are all confused about hormone replacement therapy (HRT). Originally the authors of that study thought hormone replacement would prove to have heart healthy benefits. This is not what they found, however, and they had to stop the study early. Unprecedentedly, news reports advised women to immediately stop all hormonal replacement. This mandate was the result of the increase in breast-cancer risk, heart attacks, clots in lungs, and strokes found in those who took unnatural estrogen (the brand used in the study was Premarin) and synthetic progesterone also known as progestin (the brand used in the study was Provera).

The actual medication used in the study was called Prempro and it is made up of Premarin and Provera.4 In the part of the study where women only took estrogen, they were found to be less likely to develop breast cancer, but the study's authors never addressed this discrepancy. This was an overzealous travesty keeping many women away from hormone replacement.

Since then, the Women's Health Initiative has determined that using Prempro (the combination of Premarin—horse estrogen—and the synthetic hormone Provera—a dangerous progestin) for a short duration (less than five years) and at the lowest effective dose is okay. However, they did not address the unsafe effects of the synthetic progesterone (progestin). Although they now tell women to take the lowest dose for the least amount of time, they refuse to address the use of the safe BHR that can not only overcome the symptoms of menopause, but also enhance the quality of life as women age.

The dangerous, synthetic progesterone (aka progestin or progestogen) brand name: Provera (and others—read the label and avoid progestin and progestogen), that is so often prescribed to women today causes many women to get bloated and depressed, along with increasing their risk of heart disease and cancer. Heart disease is the number one cause of death in women.

With the present hormone-prescribing scare, instead of getting the proper hormone replacement to combat the cause of their symptoms, many women receive a host of other drugs treating the individual symptoms of menopause. Sound familiar? Look in your medicine cabinet. When a woman's hormonal cascade is balanced, she is often able to discontinue many of these medications and live more comfortably.

Physicians are taught to prescribe 0.625 mg. of Premarin to women, regardless of their size or medical history. As noted, Premarin is pregnant mare's urine, aka horse estrogen. Hormone replacement therapy (HRT) is not a one-size-fits-all process. Some women need a little bit of estrogen, some women need a lot. None of them need horse estrogen, which is likely much too strong for most.

Estrogen

Estrogen is what makes a woman a woman. Without healthy estrogen, you will be dry, sad, forgetful, unmotivated, and not wanting to be sexual. So what is the problem? With the passage of time you're running on fumes of healthy estrogen. You pale in comparison to the woman you were. This change is a real physical, emotional, and psychological transformation. And the fact that estrogen is a such a no-no word in medicine puts a monkey wrench in the proverbial marital bedroom—only 20 percent of women take estrogen because when most people hear the word estrogen, the immediate thought that comes to mind is *cancer.*

Without estrogen, *you don't feel very sexual.* It really doesn't have to do with the fact that, over the passage of time your husband has become annoying. Yes, OK, so he has become annoying. But he would be less annoying if you were a properly estrogenized woman.

Without estrogen, women may have some (in extreme cases, all) of the following symptoms: aches and pains; hot flashes; temperature imbalances; night sweats; memory loss; vaginal dryness, which causes frequent urinary tract infections *and* painful sexual relations; decreased intensity of orgasms or a total inability to experience an orgasm; panic attacks; new-onset adult acne; depression; less sociability; agoraphobia; less focus on outward appearances; loss of motivation; insomnia; hair loss; carbohydrate-craving to the exclusion of nutrition; dry skin; wrinkles; headaches; and a multitude of other maladies. With this dire state of body and mind, is it any wonder that a marriage has the potential to become sexless?

But there is hope. Once you can recognize what diminished hormones are doing to you and your marriage, you can get to the properly trained doctor and receive hormones that are both safe and lifesaving.

Good Estrogen/Progesterone and Bad Estrogen/Progestin

There are many types of estrogen, both good and bad. The big point is that *good estrogen* isn't likely to cause cancer. To the contrary, good estrogen is actually good for you. When speaking of various types of estrogen, it is good to recall that there is also more than one type of progesterone. To repeat, the hormonal culprits causing the increased risk of cancer and heart disease are *synthetic* progesterone (known as progestin or progestogen), and too much exposure to the harmful estrogens.

Premarin, pregnant mare's urine that contains horse estrogen, is too strong for humans, and progestin (*synthetic* progesterone) is dangerous. Present day news reports condemning hormone replacement still use the word progesterone when they mean progestin. Progesterone is good. It is the progestin that is bad, as it constricts coronary arteries, increasing the risk for stroke and heart disease risk, and also increases the risk of cancer.

Livestock and poultry are loaded with estrogen injected by the farmers to produce plump tender animals for slaughter. That's right men, you are being feminized as you eat those juicy burgers, steaks, and BBQ chicken. And you women are getting way more estrogen that you need.

It is most likely that xenoestrogenic compounds (foreign estrogens found in our food and the environment), our obesity epidemic, and poor nutritional intake are the cause of the increase in cancer—not bio-identical estrogen.

Estrogen has a multitude of things it does (mechanisms of actions). It isn't just about hot flashes and dry vaginas anymore; it helps your bones, memory, sleep, weight, and much more. So you may be right that you require estrogen. But you don't want cancer.

Even if you had your ovaries (the main estrogen-producing glands) removed, your adrenal glands, skin, and brain can make some estrogen. And you are also getting lots of foreign estrogen in the form of xenoestrogenic compounds.

Estrogen can convert to all kinds of things with long names. 2-methyloxyestrone is the anti-carcinogenic kind of estrogen that is an antidepressant and a mood stabilizer. It hydrates the skin and vaginal vault, reverses insomnia and hot flashes, enhances libido, dilates coronary arteries, increases production of neurotransmitters, increases acetylcholine to enhance memory, builds bone, and increases collagen in skin. It is the right kind of estrogen that does not predispose you to breast cancer, but it can also convert to 4-hydroxyestrone, which is a carcinogenic type.

Taking estrogen by mouth is not natural. When you are producing your own estrogen, it is released directly into your bloodstream. When estrogen is taken by mouth, it must first be processed by your liver.

Pellets inserted under the skin slowly release estrogen for months; injections keep them level for 7–14 days, patches keep them level for 3–7 days, and topical gels or creams keep them level for 8–12 hours (creams need to be reapplied every 12 hours).

Many of the pills, patches, mists, creams, and gels (Alora, Climara, Delestrogen, Estraderm, Estrogel, Vivelle, Vivelle-DOT, and others) contain such a miniscule amount of estrogen that the results are often not therapeutic. Additionally, many women are exquisitely sensitive to the adhesive in the patches. Custom doses of bio-identical estrogen cream are effective for hot flashes, vaginal dryness, memory, a stable mood, and many of the other symptoms of menopause.

The medical environment is full of fear, which is reflected in the voices of those women required to have additional mammograms (recently downplayed as diagnostic tools), ultrasounds, or MRIs of their breasts at the sign of the slightest lump, bump, or irregularity of the breast. Some are even required to have a needle excision localized biopsy. After prescribing bio-identical hormone replacement therapy for over two decades, I (RM) have only had one woman receive a breast cancer diagnosis that was a non-invasive type.

There are so many ways to reduce your chances of getting breast, or any other kind of cancer. Much of it has to do with lifestyle changes. The choice to be healthy or not is yours.

Why Are Newborns Born with High Levels of Bad Estrogen?

The umbilical cords of newborn baby boys and girls are being tested and they are finding that, amazingly, newborns already have high levels of Bisphenol-A (BPA). This is a plastic—a synthetic form of estrogen. These toxic plastics are environmental contaminants and they seem to be everywhere.[5]

Gender Identity Disorder

Can you even guess why there is a new diagnosis in pediatrics called gender identity disorder (GID)? Those who seek transgender surgery are different, genetically and neurologically, and scientists have speculated that environmental changes have altered the genetic structure. It is thought that estrogens, the harmful ones, are one of the reasons for this.

A Petrochemical Sea of Xenoestrogens

You have estrogen even if you are not taking estrogen. This is because estrogens, real and fake, are components of many products. Xenoestrogens are synthetic fake estrogens derived from many sources that everyone comes in contact with in the normal course of events. These sources include petroleum oil, plastics, medicine, clothing, food, soap, pesticides, herbicides, spermicides, condoms, breakdown products of surfactants commonly used in detergents, cosmetics, and even perfumes. One example of the damaging effects of environmental exposure to synthetic xenoestrogenic estrogen is that male alligators in Florida are being born with questionable female genitalia. And girls as young as eight are getting their first period from all the bad estrogen they are exposed to in their diet and environment.

Phytoestrogens

Some plants produce estrogen-like substances called phytoestrogens. The main dietary sources of phytoestrogens are soybeans and soy products, but flaxseeds also contain large amounts of them and they are found in high-fiber foods, such as cereal brans and beans. When it comes to estrogen, it's a bit like Goldilocks—you want your estrogen levels to be *just right*. This is why testing your hormone levels is so important, even if you have no symptoms yet.

Estrogen Can Convert to Healthy or Carcinogenic Types

For those who think estrogen is always bad, you need to know that there are many, many of kinds of estrogen, including the good kind mentioned above, 2-methoxyestrone, which is anti-carcinogenic (but not 4-hydroxyestrone, which *is* carcinogenic). Another kind of estrogen called 16 alpha hydroxyestrone is also carcinogenic. So when you hear the news telling you to take HRT for a short time, or not to take HRT at all, it's important to know which kind, and how much estrogen and progesterone they're talking about.

Three Major Types of Estrogen

The estrogen story expands in scope because you should realize that while there are hundreds of types of estrogen, humans have three major types.

Estrone—E1 is in fat cells, so possessing too much fat predisposes you to breast cancer. However, with minor lifestyle modifications, E1 can convert to the more beneficial E3.

Estradiol—E2 is the predominant estrogen that's made in a woman's twenties. This is the strongest, but not the worst—E2 converting to 16 hydroxyestrone is the worst.

Estriol—E3 is the estrogen made during pregnancy and it is the weakest estrogen. This pregnancy estrogen is thought to be protective in that it does not stimulate breast tissue to grow and is not able to stimulate the endometrium (uterine wall) to thicken. This weak estrogen is anti-carcinogenic. This is one reason why women who have multiple pregnancies have a lower incidence of breast cancer. In connection with this, note that fewer and fewer children are being born. Could this have something to do with the increase in breast cancer?

Have your estradiol levels (the good estrogen of youth) tested, and if needed, take estrogen in small (*physiologic*) amounts to prevent heart disease and Alzheimer's, two major maladies that can affect people as they age.

Estrogen Delivery Parentally

Parenteral means that the delivery system of taking a drug is not by mouth. Parenteral includes transdermal (through the skin) patches, transdermal creams, vaginal creams, injections, and pellets placed under the skin. In every one of these systems, the first pass of the hormone is on the tissues of the body, not the liver.

Estrogen and Your Diet

There are dietary ways to limit or enhance the amount of estrogen you have in your body. Be aware that extremes of any type are not good for you and you should avoid extremes with dietary/estrogen matters. If you do wish to boost or lower your estrogen by diet, here are some ideas.

Foods that increase your own estrogen or contain high levels of estrogen that are absorbed into the body include *cultured* and *fermented* soybean products, such as tempeh, natto, pickled tofu, miso, and soy sauce—not soy milk, soy peanuts, soy protein bars, protein shakes, or the multitude of soy products found everywhere. The fermented soy is actually healthy while regular soy products decrease thyroid levels and have metabolites that inhibit enzymatic pathways. There is so much controversy about the benefits versus the risks associated with various types of soy that it is best to use moderation in their consumption until definite answers become available.

Other foods that increase estrogen are apples, beets, berries, chickpeas (hummus), eggplant, flaxseeds, garlic, hops, licorice, lima beans, oats, papaya, parsley, plums, pomegranates, potatoes, tomatoes, and yams. While alcohol decreases many hormones, it actually increases estradiol. Eat lean protein and foods low in fat and high in fiber to increase estrogen levels.

Foods that inhibit estrogen production/activity include broccoli, cabbage, cauliflower, corn, grapes, green beans, melons, pineapple, squash, white flour, and white rice.

If you are trying to keep your estrogen balanced, there's no need to either avoid these foods or eat them to abundance, just avoid excesses. The best way to tell if your estrogen and other hormone levels are healthy is by getting a blood test. Your doctor should then integrate the laboratory results with how you look, combined with your complaints. Your estrogen level is unique. The lab result is just a reference point.

Again—Does Estrogen Cause Breast Cancer?

It is sad that people think in such a linear Newtonian-physics way and relegate estrogen to being the premier road to developing breast cancer. As has been pointed out, estrogen-like foreign chemicals called xenoestrogenic compounds found in the environment and food supply lodge in your fatty tissue. This xenoestrogenic, fake estrogen does increase the risk of breast cancer. Being overweight/obese increases the risk of breast cancer because so much estrogen is retained in fat tissue.

Anti-Carcinogenic Substances
that Help Prevent Breast Cancer

- Progesterone—real progesterone, not the progestins and progestogens found in Prempro, Provera, and oral contraceptives.

- Testosterone—vitally important. Testosterone prevents the stimulation of breast cells by xenoestrogenic estrogenic compounds, synthetic prescribed estrogen such as Premarin, and synthetic progestins such as Provera. Testosterone is prescribed to treat breast cancer patients in other countries.

- Estriol—the weak estrogen produced predominately during pregnancy.

- B_{12}—As methylcobalamin (not cyanocobalamin or hydroxocobalamin), this vitamin, administered sublingually or by injection, converts estrogen to healthy 2-methoxyestrogen.

- Iodine—this stimulates the metabolism of estradiol and estrone into estriol and forms iodolipids (fats combined with iodine) that kill many types of breast cancer.

- 2 methoxyestrogen—a healthy form of estrogen.

- Flax oil and lignans (fiber)—enhance the conversion of estrogen to 2-hydroxyestrogen.

- Indole 3-carbinol (I3C)—enhances the conversion of estrogen to 2-hydroxyestrogen.

- Increased ratio of 2-hydroxyestrogen to 16-hydroxyestrogen.

- Vitamin D—presently known to turn off sixty-three cell lines of cancer.

- DHEA (dehydroepiandosterone)—decreases G6PD, glucose 6 phosphate dehydrogenase, which feeds anaerobic energy to cancer cells that thrive and replicate in non-oxygen environments.

- Melatonin—the natural sleep hormone.

Carcinogenic Substances That Can Cause Breast Cancer

- Synthetic progestins and progestogens—found in Provera and birth control pills.

- Medroxyprogesterone—a synthetic progesterone found in Prempro.

- Too much adrenaline/stress—you cannot methylate your estrogen to a healthy form if it is methylating your increased stress hormone—adrenaline. To prevent breast cancer, decrease the stressors in your life. Consider doing some form of meditation. This may be accomplished with traditional mediation techniques or by using emWave technology by Heart Math made for your computer. The program will teach you how to control your heartbeats with breathing.

- Toxic food, toxic hunger—cravings that are not hunger.

- Fat—and not knowing how many pounds of fat you have. It's not about losing weight, it's about losing fat, and doing it slowly because it is toxic and as it is shed, it releases those toxins.

- Insufficient progesterone, estriol, B^{12}, iodine, testosterone, DHEA, vitamin D, melatonin, and indole 3-carbinol—deficiencies of these are unhealthy and potentially carcinogenic.

- Radiation—in the form of x-rays, mammograms, CT scans.

- Estrogen taken by mouth—estrogen should never be taken by mouth as it accumulates in the liver and causes problems.

- Longtime use of oral contraceptives—they contain synthetic hormones.

- Synthetic estrogen—it's too strong.

- Alcohol—in excess.

- Smoking.

- Animal protein and dairy—The China Study authors' concluded that those populations consuming lots of animal-based foods are more likely to die from Western diseases, such as cancer and coronary disease. The opposite was true for populations eating more plant foods.[6]

- Too little exercise—exercise sends more oxygen to all your cells and oxygen kills cancer cells.

- Too much sugar—sugar helps cancer grow.

- Acidic foods—the American diet is acidic and unhealthy. A whole food, plant-based diet rich in volume and nutrients is alkaline and healthy.

Who's Going To Treat You?

Women usually expect their gynecologists to be specialists in hormone replacement therapy (HRT). But gynecologists are trained as surgeons, so most are not familiar with HRT, and even fewer understand BHRT. My (RM) women patients tell me they don't get much information from their gynecologists, though they do get prescriptions for dangerous synthetic hormones because that's what the pharmacy salespeople promote. If women don't like what they hear at the gynecologist, they then go to an endocrinologist who, they discover, really only treats diabetes and thyroid disorders (endocrinologists tell me the ovaries are not their turf). It seems nobody wants to claim responsibility for hormone replacement, or the training is lax in certain areas. Women intuitively know they need hormones, but they have fears. Welcome the integrative medicine specialist who actually trains in tendering the entire hormonal cascade.

If your doctor is not well-versed in the subject of hormone replacement therapy (and many are not), the first thing he/she will usually say when you bring up the subject will be a simple statement that it is dangerous. More specifically, supporting the old school of thought, she/he will likely tell you it can cause breast or ovarian cancer.

It is known that certain cancers tend to grow faster with exposure to high doses of estrogen, especially when this estrogen comes from external sources called xenoestrogens (from plastics, chemicals, and food sources injected with estrogen). This has all been outlined at length in this book, and now that you are armed with the facts, and understand that you are seeking bio-identical hormones, never synthetic, or animal-derived, hormones, and that your blood and urine levels must be monitored. Now you are in a position to take control of your future and seek the right doctor to assist you.

While hormone replacement should be for everyone, it isn't. Who wouldn't want to slow the aging process, live a more vital life, enhance their relationships, and extend sexual prowess into old age? If offered this package, who would turn it down?

The main reason hormone replacement isn't more actively employed is due to the limited number of practitioners who have the knowledge, time, or desire to engage in such practice. There is also fear associated with hormones and their perceived link to cancer. And finally, you don't see everyone flocking to this form of therapy due to the cost. It is not covered by most medical insurance, and most people don't have the money to seek the treatment on their own.

Medical insurance covers acute conditions that, if left untreated, cause pain, suffering, and death, but when it comes to issues revolving around quality of life, there is just not enough money to go around in a society that fears playing with *the natural order of things*. However, this fear is unfounded, as all medicine and every form of treatment alter the natural order of things.

Since at this time insurance usually doesn't cover BHRT, it is up to the individual to decide if it will be a priority for them. If it just isn't feasible for you, there are still many other suggestions in this book that will help the individual and the sexless marriage.

Bio-Identical Hormone Replacement Therapy—BHRT

Medical doctors who are trained by European endocrinologists prescribe hormones that are biochemically identical to the estrogen, progesterone, and testosterone women make in their twenties. These biochemically identical hormones are given in individually tailored low doses that are monitored by blood tests for hormone levels.

Bio-identical hormone replacement therapy (BHRT) has been prescribed in Europe for more than sixty-five years, with no increase in breast cancer. But European physicians do not prescribe horse estrogen or synthetic progesterone.

BHRT is recognized for safely resolving the multitudinous symptoms of menopause and perimenopause—hot flashes, night sweats, temperature imbalances, loss of libido, vaginal dryness, difficulty achieving orgasm or decreased intensity of orgasm, depression, weight gain, mood swings, irritability, memory loss, hair loss, myalgias (muscle pain), fibromyalgia, and insomnia with difficulty getting or remaining asleep (or both).

Prescribing hormones is highly individualized and is done only after an extensive menstrual and reproductive history has been taken and laboratory studies have been done to learn what is deficient.

Even after they've seen other doctors, to date no women have ever come to this office (RM) with a proper hormonal workup based on blood or urine testing. They have had their FSH and LH levels done, but all this indicates is that a woman is menopausal. A more complete workup should include estradiol (one of the three types of natural estrogen) on day 12, progesterone on day 21 if they are still menstruating, cortisol, DHEA-S, pregnenolone, thyroid studies, and free testosterone (women need a tiny bit of testosterone), among others.

Testosterone Replacement

Replacing testosterone in women has been an enlightening experience for me (RM). Women who never liked sex, and I mean never, suddenly realized they were sexual beings. Other women, who were too nice and tried to make everyone happy, found they had a voice. Women who were lean but flabby were able to build muscle. Women slept better. Husbands have been pleasantly surprised by the results. For some men, it's like having their wives returned to them. Yes, women need a little testosterone.

Symptoms of testosterone overdose are not a hoarse voice and a beard as many women fear. Excessive testosterone replacement in women results in oily hair and skin, acne, chin hairs, and sparse hair around the lips (you get unwanted hair growth all in the wrong places). In over twenty years, I have seen two women experience clitoral or vulvar hypertrophy (enlargement). If a woman is applying a judicious individually tailored dose of testosterone and she is properly treated with estrogen first, she will experience only the positive benefits.

LINDA AND TOM'S LIBIDOS

(RM) Linda, married to Tom for twenty-seven years, was a patient who sought counsel with me for BHRT. With treatment, Linda slowly emerged into the woman she once was. I was thrilled to see her redevelop into a vibrant woman who could sleep, think, maintain imperturbable equanimity in the face of adversity, and desire sex with her husband. After years of living in a relatively sexless marriage, Linda actually felt sexual again. She wanted to be with her husband. With Linda's long lost libido found, there was one little issue to be addressed—her husband Tom. His libido was still long lost. Linda was on the case.

Tom was fifty-five, overweight, and on multiple medications for high cholesterol, hypertension, and diabetes. Linda had expected the outside of Tom to change with time, but she had always thought Tom would be the same man inside. But where was the man she had married? Tom used to have strong opinions about life and people. Tom used to have an edge. Tom used to laugh. Tom used to exercise and have some muscle. Tom used to get excited about things. Tom used to be alive. Even though Tom was only two years older than Linda, he seemed to be much older inside. And Linda wanted to have sex with Tom again. Linda still loved Tom.

The following scenario is a frequent one in my medical practice. Linda noticed men in my waiting room and asked if I also have men patients. I replied that one-third of my practice is men, and many predict that in future years I may see more men than women. I briefly explained that reviving a man hormonally is multifaceted and involves much more than rubbing some testosterone gel on his chest.

So Linda asked Tom to seek medical counsel with me. Crankily, Tom said, "I don't need testosterone and that other stuff she does. Anyway, my urologist tested my testosterone and said it was normal for my age. That TV commercial is a bunch of crap. Anyway, testosterone causes prostate cancer." In spite of this, Tom eventually became a quasi-reluctant new patient.

Over time Tom and Linda's marriage had devolved from feeling passion for life and each other to a marriage where they quietly existed as robotic housemates. They developed their little routines.

They remembered how their marriage used to have a bounding pulse and a purpose. The pulse of their marriage was still audible, but it was weak. They quietly lived with each other in what seemed to be solitary confinement, with occasional time off for good behavior when they went to work.

Tom and Linda were rational people. They did realize that marriage, including romantic interludes, would be redefined after the children arrived. But what they didn't expect was that sex would become lifeless and rare.

Tom didn't talk to his wife about why they didn't have sex. Being sort of sexless was merely accepted. He didn't ask or tell anyone about his sexless marriage. He thought it was him. Then he told me that maybe it was his wife, because on the rare occasion they tried to have sex she would be dry, and sex would be uncomfortable. Then Tom admitted he was often embarrassed because getting and keeping an erection was hit or miss. The little blue pill helped, but not always, only sometimes.

Tom and Linda were seeing separate therapists to discuss issues with their children and work. Occasionally, they would see their individual therapists together. Actually, when I counted, there were over *ten* physicians who cared for Tom and Linda. But not one of them had ever asked Tom, or Linda, about their sexuality. For these doctors, Tom and Linda's marital love life was not part of the medical puzzle, which I found amazing. Then I remembered that medical training did not include sexology, the replacement of declining hormones(ology), advice on how to be healthy(ology), weight loss(ology), or nutritional biochemistry(ology).

At my suggestion, Tom did some reading about how he didn't have to age inside as fast as he was aging outside. He realized the game wasn't over. After the correct hormonal panel was completed and interpreted, Tom started replacing waning hormones. He started thinking about sex again. Our consultations about how to bring out the old Tom with social dominance and virility began in earnest. Linda and Tom were finally back as a couple helped by a little judiciously administered testosterone.

Diagnostic Tests and Related Methods
to Evaluate Women

This section is especially beneficial for your physician.

The tests required for evaluating women include: FSH/LH, estradiol, progesterone, sex hormone-binding globulin, free testosterone, cortisol, DHEA-S, TSH (thyroid-stimulating hormone), T3, T4, free T3, free T4, reverse T3, antithyroglobulin antibodies, antithyroperoxidase antibodies.

A thorough history, including the dates of menarche, any pregnancy, any infertility, and any STDs must be taken. The doctor needs to know: Does the patient have a libido? Does she masturbate? Can she reach climax? If not, did she ever reach climax? Does she know that only 10–15 percent of women can achieve penis in vagina orgasms? What are her major stressors (inattentive husband, aging parents, unruly offspring, family issues, job stressors, addiction)? What medications, if any, is she presently taking? Can she sleep? Does she dream? Does she poop? Does she worry? Does she have a passion for something, anything?

Following the extensive workup, the protocol for treatment includes replacing, in low physiologic doses, all the hormones that are produced in the anterior pituitary. The doctor should start with estrogen, progesterone (not progestins or progestogens), and intra-vaginal estriol for vaginal dryness.

RESTORING CHARLOTTE'S JOY IN LIFE

(RM) Charlotte's first period occurred at age sixteen (she is now fifty years old), her menses were never regular, and she would go as long as six months between cycles. As a result, oral contraceptives were started at seventeen that resulted in regular menses and continued for over thirty years. There were minor periods of time when she stopped using the pill—for five miscarriages and two live births. A fertility workup for Charlotte and her husband was negative (meaning there was no problem). Oral contraceptives were discontinued three years ago when her husband had a vasectomy.

For the past three years, Charlotte's menses have been highly irregular. Sometimes she experiences her period in sixty days, and then has another twelve days later. Some of them are quite heavy, and some are so light that she wonders if she really had a period. Sleep is in the past. Headaches are a new symptom on the horizon and are worse prior to her period. Sex is painful, secondary to dryness. Orgasms are nearly impossible even after liberal lubrication. If an orgasm does occur, Charlotte asks herself, "Was that it?"

She remembers seeing the humor in life in the past, but now life just seems like something to get through. Her previous sense of joy, which was contagious, is gone. She asks me, "Will I ever feel the same again?" I wholeheartedly assure her that she will. A pelvic ultrasound (transvaginal, to visualize the ovaries, and transabdominal, to visualize her uterus) confirmed my suspicion that Charlotte has PCOS (polycystic ovarian syndrome). This is why her periods were always so irregular or absent, and this is what contributed to her multiple miscarriages. Historically, Charlotte was low in estrogen and even lower in progesterone. The hormones in the oral contraceptives she had taken for years simply mimicked pregnancy, prevented ovulation, and worsened the hormonal milieu.

Blood tests confirmed that Charlotte was entering menopause, as the markers for this transition, her FSH and LH levels, were high. Her levels of estradiol, progesterone, SHBG, free testosterone, and multiple thyroid tests were abnormal and not in balance.

A prescription for bio-identical transdermal progesterone taken on days 15–25 helped calm Charlotte and restore her sleep. Progesterone (not progestin or progestogen, which constrict coronary arteries and increase the risk of a heart attack, stroke, and breast cancer) also helped produce regular monthly cycles. Later, her sleep improved even more when the transdermal application was changed to capsules on days 10–25 taken at bedtime.

Unlike estrogen, progesterone can be taken in capsule form, which actually changes to a molecule similar to a tranquilizer and often results in baby sleep—Charlotte was slowly weaned off her tranquilizer and her sleeping pill, both of which only serve to disrupt deep sleep.

Charlotte received a low-dose prescription for bio-identical testosterone, which was applied once a day to the inner vulva, the clitoral hood, and sometimes the intra-vaginal G spot (she was given a tutorial on where her G spot was located) and all of this helped to restore her libido a bit. With the additional combination of having her testosterone restored, discontinuing her second antidepressant and changing the first antidepressant to one without negative sexual side effects, Charlotte began to have sexual dreams again. On follow-up visits, she reported that her interest and ability to reach climax was restored.

After two months on the bio-identical hormones, Charlotte lost ten pounds with no changes in her eating habits. There was still much to teach her regarding how, where, when, and why to eat, along with behavioral changes, all of which resulted in further weight loss. For added benefit, exercising by doing something enjoyable was incorporated into her schedule at least four times a week.

Detailed instruction on how to eat (thorough chewing) and the addition of a low dose of betaine hydrochloride (stomach acid) insured the absorption of quality nutrition and supplementation. The pulling on tendons and ligaments during exercise also helped to absorb the twenty-two minerals that are required to build new bone.

The bisphosphonate, bone-building medication was discontinued, secondary to no improvement upon reviewing Charlotte's previous DEXA scans and her concerns about a possible femur fracture and jaw infection, which had been recently reported in the media.

She was also educated about the inappropriateness of too much calcium. Calcium and magnesium need to be given in a one-to-one ratio, but to date, no patient has ever brought in a multi-mineral formulation with that ratio.

Her upper and lower endoscopies were negative, so her antacid was discontinued, leading to even more new bone growth. A thorough testing of her thyroid revealed a problem that contributed to her hair loss, low energy, and difficulty sleeping. Treatment with low-dose, sustained-release T4/T3 helped resolve her symptoms.

Blood studies showed that Charlotte was grossly deficient in vitamin D, zinc, red blood cells, magnesium, B12, and folic acid, plus
she had elevated iron levels. Her potassium was low and her triglycerides were high due to her previous nutrient-deficient diet. The
revised eating and supplement program I provided helped further
wean Charlotte off the remaining antidepressant, which, by the way,
wasn't working. With the addition of exercise and doing something
she enjoyed once a day, her previous joy for life returned, slowly. She
is now a shining example of how joy can be restored.

The Effects of Bone Loss (Osteoporosis) on a Relationship

Osteoporosis affects more women than men, and although bone loss
may not have specific sexual side effects (no one ever said a dowager's
hump was sexy), this is a good time to discuss it, because the effects of
brittle and/or broken bones can make sexual activity risky and painful.

Bone deterioration is a silent disease. You don't want to find that
your broken bones and the attendant pain that's keeping you from
sexual activity were, unbeknownst to you, brewing for many years.
Prevention is the best medicine, which entails staying away from
those undertakings that break down bone. This list includes alcohol,
carbonated beverages, excess protein, inactivity, smoking, steroids,
stress, acid blockers, too much calcium, and the phosphates in sodas
and most meat—even cancer can be included here.

The Prevention and Reversal of Osteoporosis

Osteoporosis is preventable when you become involved in your most
precious acquisition—a healthy body.

At about age thirty-five, women start to lose 1.5 percent of their
bone mass per year.[7] During the formative years, they make deposits
in the way of minerals (calcium, also magnesium, boron, zinc, selenium, copper)—twenty-two minerals are needed to make new bone.[8]
And, interestingly, during that time the body is able to make some

vitamins and amino acids, but not one single mineral. Now, at age thirty-five, the woman's body starts making bone withdrawals.

All forty-something women (and most men) need a baseline DEXA scan (dual energy x-ray absorbtiometry), which is an x-ray of your lumbar spine and hips (have them x-ray both hips). It has been my experience (RM) that the heel scan provides minimal information, plus some patients have osteoporosis in one hip and not the other. What if the wrong hip got x-rayed?

The DEXA report gives two scores, a T score and a Z score. The T score compares your bones to thirty-year-olds. The Z score compares your bones to people your age. Normally, DEXA scans are not ordered until a woman breaks a bone (stepping off a curb and breaking an ankle, for example), or when a person is in their seventies. Too late. An ounce of prevention is not worth a pound of cure, but tons and tons of cure.

The bottom line: you want to build bone. You want to have a positive T score, no bone loss. You want bone to be built faster than it is being broken down. If the score is negative, this means you have lost bone. If the score is −2.5 or less, then you have osteoporosis (think of bones that look like honeycombs). A score of −1 up to −2.5 means you have osteopenia, mild bone loss. Not osteoporosis yet, but your bones are journeying toward osteoporosis land. Not good. Integrative medicine is optimistic medicine, so the good news is that bone loss is preventable and reversible.

You may want to check out Dr. Alan Gaby's groundbreaking book, *Preventing and Reversing Osteoporosis.*[9] Unfortunately, the material in this book is not taught in conventional medical training, as those schools mainly teach how to prescribe FDA-approved drugs called bisphosphonates which help, but have a number of associated risks, including jawbone infections that don't heal well.

Minerals for Osteoporosis

There are ways to maintain and rebuild bone and avoid taking prescription medication. Calcium, yes, but there are twenty-two minerals that make new bone. Certain types of calcium are better absorbed. For example, calcium citrate is better absorbed if you are not producing enough stomach acid, as in patients taking antacids. If you take your calcium with meals so your stomach acid is flowing, and if you don't take antacids, the cheaper calcium carbonate works well. The calcium/magnesium ratio of my patients is closer to 1/1. (RM)

Hormone Replacement Therapy (HRT) for Osteoporosis

Please be aware that what you are hearing in the media is about synthetic HRT. Real estrogen helps to prevent further bone breakdown, but does not help rebuild bone. Real progesterone, melatonin, DHEA, testosterone, and properly absorbed minerals are what help build new bone.

Strength Training Exercise for Osteoporosis

This form of exercise helps build bone. You don't need to live in the gym. Twenty minutes, twice a week is all you need. Have someone teach you to do men's pushups. Most of my women patients are able to do half a pushup their first try.

RESTORED TO MENTAL AND PHYSICAL HEALTH

(RM) Cynthia S. is a fifty-year-old woman who told me she couldn't sleep, and as a result experienced debilitating fatigue, which then led to a host of other symptoms. The five specialists she saw before me sent her for psychiatric counseling. As a result, Cynthia is now on an antidepressant and a second psychiatric medication because the first antidepressant isn't working. She is also on a beta blocker for her heart palpitations after the cardiologist performed a complete cardiac workup, which was negative. At 5'2" she now weighs 180 lbs and reports a sixty-pound weight gain without changing her eating habits.

I prescribed a low-dose bio-identical transdermal, Biestrogen (a compounded formula of 20 percent estradiol and 80 percent estriol), that was rubbed on the soft part of the upper arms for twenty-five days, morning and night, and it restored her estrogen to normal levels. This resulted in a regular menstrual bleed every month because estrogen is required to create a lining in your uterus. No estrogen, no menstrual bleed. When too much estrogen builds up, however, you have a heavy menstrual bleed. The estrogen restored hydration of Cynthia's vaginal cells and sex was no longer painful. There was a noticeable improvement in the hydration of her skin as well, which was an added aesthetic benefit.

Additional sexual therapy for Cynthia included a prescription of a vaginal cream containing sildenafil (Viagra), arginine, and amino-phyline to increase blood flow to the clitoral hood. As the medical studies suggest, low-dose intra-vaginal DHEA (dehydroepiandoste-rone) suppositories helped increase the intensity of the climax.[10] She was advised to read *The Kama Sutra* and *The Joy of Sex* to reignite relations with her beloved. There was also a discussion of the use of sexual toys, clitoral vs. vaginal orgasms, and sundry other discussions regarding intimate communion.

A DEXA scan showed that Cynthia was nearing a diagnosis of osteoporosis. Repeat studies showed there was much improvement in her bone thickness after resuming her hormones, taking the correct twenty-two minerals to build bone (not twenty-two bottles of supplements), increasing her vitamin D to 5000 IUs a day, and getting monthly injections of vitamin D (vitamin D is required for minerals to be absorbed into bone), along with periodic blood testing of 25-hydroxy vitamin D.

DHEA

DHEA (dehydroepiandrosterone) is placed in this chapter on women's hormones though it is just as important for men for its role in human sexuality and health.

DHEA is a hormone produced by your adrenal glands. It can do many things on its own. However, since it can be converted to testosterone or estradiol, it must be used carefully and only with medical supervision. It is considered an androgen (a steroid hormone), which is naturally produced by both men and women. DHEA is the most abundant hormone in your body and resides in every single one of your trillion cells.

The list of health benefits afforded with *physiologic* (small dose) replacement of DHEA is scientifically clear and impressive. For starters, DHEA decreases abdominal fat, enhances the libido and sexual function, thickens skin, boosts immunity, and is neuroprotective. DHA is often confused with DHEA. DHA (docosahexaenoic acid) is not a hormone; rather it is a one of the omega-3 fatty acids that reduces inflammation and strengthens brain and eye function.

With aging, those who have very low levels of DHEA combined with a precipitous rise in cortisol and insulin are more likely to develop dementia. The meteoric rise in insulin with poor diet and aging is being called type 3 diabetes, and is associated with an increased risk of Alzheimer's disease.[11] There are those who now suggest that Alzheimer's disease is actually a form of insulin resistance in the brain. The neuroprotective (brain-protective) effects of DHEA are profoundly beneficial to aging well, since there is ultimately nothing as important as slowing down the aging of the brain.

You will need a prescription for the DHEA-S blood test, and testing means continued monitoring to make sure all the hormones remain in balance. The most effective way to take DHEA is by mouth with food.

There is a form of DHEA called 7-keto DHEA that does not convert to testosterone or estrogen, and as such, it is not risky to take from a sex hormone point of view. Since it does not convert to the stronger hormones that have so much to do with sex, you won't see those kinds of benefits. 7-keto DHEA is best known for its ability to help with weight loss (it burns up fat), as well as help with the immune system (it fights off infections.)

DHEA's Role in Sexuality and Health

The dramatic drop in DHEA levels observed as people age parallels the development of degenerative problems, including a decline of the immune system, clogged blood vessels, thinning bones, mental decline, depression, and the increased risk of cancer.

DHEA has been shown in studies and in human trials to increase women's libidos and strength of climax. For the men, nearly all the focus on hormones and erectile function has been with testosterone, but DHEA plays a major role as well—both testosterone and DHEA may require replacement in physiologic doses for optimal libido and erectile function. As noted, DHEA may convert into testosterone or estrogen, which is why symptoms may occur when too much is taken. In men, these symptoms include oily skin and hair, and breast tenderness. Ongoing blood testing is required to make sure all hormones levels remain balanced.

DHEA peaks around the age of twenty, you have one-half that amount by your fourth decade, and by the time you are eighty, you will be running on fumes.[12] This is typical for the natural aging process, which is inextricably tied to a decrease in beneficial hormones—DHEA, estrogen, growth hormone, melatonin, progesterone, and testosterone—that is accompanied by an increase in such harmful hormones as cortisol and insulin.

In young men, the daily production of DHEA is 30 milligrams, and in young women, it is 20 milligrams a day. Diets rich in sugar, sweets, cereals, and grain decrease DHEA levels.

For women, the symptoms of a DHEA deficiency include clitoral atrophy, the loss of pubic fat (Mont de Venus), the loss of underarm, pubic, and leg hair, dry eyes and skin, and a decreased, or absent, libido, usually accompanied by decreased or absent orgasms.

Women must have enough estrogen to balance DHEA (and testosterone) or symptoms of an overdose will manifest. For women, the symptoms of excessive DHEA are similar to those for men—oily skin and hair, and breast tenderness if DHEA is converted to estrogen.

While DHEA is readily available over the counter in many countries, it can wreak havoc if you take too much. If you are interested in trying DHEA, you should really seek the medical counsel of a physician trained and knowledgeable in bio-identical hormone replacement therapy.

Oxytocin

Oxytocin is another hormone that is important for both men and women, though it is more often thought of as the hormone that helps the uterus contract during childbirth. In *Passion, Sex and Long Life—The Incredible Oxytocin Adventure*,[13] Dr. Thierry Hertoghe calls oxytocin the love hormone. Oxytocin is released from the brain during sexual activities and especially upon orgasm. The result is that the couple feels bonded and close.

In Europe, oxytocin is prescribed to enhance sexual function for women who take twenty minutes or longer to have a weak climax. To determine who needs this type of intervention, a detailed sexual history must be taken, a rare occurrence since many American doctors don't even ask if the patient is still sexual.

Oxytocin increases vaginal lubrication, increases uterine and vaginal contractions at orgasm, decreases adrenaline, and decreases carbohydrate craving. Women and men who take SSRI antidepressants, such as Prozac, Celexa, Zoloft, and others, often report that it takes hours to climax and then they wonder if they really did. SSRI antidepressants lower oxytocin, block the action of oxytocin, and usually prevent climax. Anti-estrogen drugs also decrease oxytocin with the resultant decreased frequency and intensity of climax.

Women need four hormones for sexual arousal: estradiol (estrogen), testosterone, MSH (see below) and oxytocin. On the occasions that estradiol and testosterone don't improve sexual arousal, oxytocin and/or MSH can be prescribed.

MSH

Melanocyte stimulating hormone (MSH) is produced in the pituitary gland and it stimulates the production of melanin, which is responsible for the color of skin and hair. This means you will get tan without the sun when supplementing with this hormone, but that is not its intended use. MSH is prescribed by European endocrinologists to enhance sexual arousal, inhibit appetite, and enhance a natural tan.

MSH is administered by injection and should be done under the guidance of your physician because too much may lower your own cortisol to dangerous levels and cause age spots to darken.

Postmenopausal women treated with MSH tell me (RM), "It was like when we were dating in our 30s. I was 100 percent into it. I was in the mood and I started initiating again. I was focused on sex, and was able to reach climax easily and with more intensity, like when I was young. I wasn't thinking of anything else."

If partners still like each other, just imagine how many marriages would be enhanced and possibly saved by prescribing low doses of bio-identical estradiol, testosterone, oxytocin, and MSH. Saving marriages is paramount because no one else is going to know your history and love your children the way your partner does.

Non-Hormonal Treatment for Menopause?

There are many estrogen products that are applied topically for vaginal dryness (Estrace, Estring, Femring, and Vagifem among them). They were developed with the idea of limiting the amount of estrogen, as always suggesting the unproven notion that estrogen is detrimental. While these topical products have not been studied as much as estrogen pills, there is still the chance that they can get into the bloodstream, and that fosters an unfounded fear. As a result, medical studies continue to search for the perfect non-hormone remedy for the myriad deleterious symptoms of menopause.

The FDA has approved the first non-hormonal therapy for moderate to severe hot flashes associated with menopause. This drug, Brisdelle, is actually a lower dose of the SSRI antidepressant Paxil. Why would anyone want to take a medication that has a list of adverse reactions that include sexual problems, manic episodes, seizures, suicidal thoughts, and more? While bio-identical estrogen safely provides relief for the growing list of symptoms that result from hormone imbalances, the media's fear-based stance against estrogen continues, and this relegates you to a medication that is going to make you feel worse than you already do.

Hopefully the adverse effects of Brisdelle are not typical. However, it now appears that the FDA wanted to offer a non-hormone alternative for women, even to the point of ignoring their own advisory committee, which concluded that Brisdelle did not provide any meaningful improvement over a placebo.[14]

Osphena (ospemifene) has been approved by the FDA as the first non-estrogen pill to treat moderate to severe dyspareunia (pain during intercourse) due to menopause. Ironically though, it may increase hot flashes. What a tradeoff.

Ospemifene is known as a selective estrogen receptor modulator (SERM). This class of drugs behaves like estrogen in some tissues while blocking estrogen in others. For example, the SERM tamoxifen (Nolvadex, Soltamox) and toremifene (Fareston) are FDA approved to treat breast cancer by blocking estrogen in the breast although both drugs can cause uterine cancer and blood clots by acting like regular estrogen. The SERM raloxifene (Evista) is approved for osteoporosis, but does nothing to prevent breast cancer, yet still has the potential to cause blood clots.

You have to wonder why anyone would want to take drugs with unknown outcomes when there is bio-identical estrogen (not horse estrogen or synthetics) available to remedy such symptoms of menopause as painful sex. According to Public Citizen, there is much that remains unknown about the safety of these new drugs.[15]

7

All About Men—
Male Sexuality

IT'S IMPORTANT TO EXPLORE THE ROOT CAUSES OF WHY MEN STOP having sex. There are many, and they include disease and health issues, obesity, chronic pain, depression, low self-esteem, low libido, low hormones, erectile dysfunction, premature ejaculation, stress, drug and/or alcohol abuse, smoking, medications (especially antide-pressants, anti-anxiety drugs, and blood-pressure medication), guilt, shame, sexual abuse, post-traumatic stress disorder . . . and one very big reason—an unwilling partner. Interestingly, many of these causes are interconnected and can be a result of the biggest reason of all—low hormone levels in either or both partners.

The Vicious Cycle

Most who experience the natural decline of vital chemicals produced by the body never see the connection. They live dysfunctional lives that affect not only themselves, but also their entire family. Most doctors watch as old people wither away. They merely look on as the skin of older people gets so thin that a simple bump on the edge of a table requires stitches, a fall breaks hips and other bones that then put them in a deathbed where pneumonia ultimately kills them. Is this natural? Well, in a way, yes, but it doesn't have to be that way.

Male Sexuality—General Information

Male sexuality peaks at about eighteen, while female sexuality usually peaks at around thirty. (*See* Chapter 9 regarding sexual peak.) However, more and more female patients tell me (RM) that they found their sexual purpose and a new joy for life in their fifties and sixties. Men need to take advantage of this newfound sexuality and engage with their willing partners rather than sit on the sidelines letting all good things pass. If they have lost interest in sex, they should do whatever is necessary to get back in the game.

It isn't always true that men in hormonal decline can't have sex. To the contrary, they may engage regularly, either alone or with a mate. What they often find with advancing age may not necessarily define full-blown erectile dysfunction, but rather less interest in sex and the need for more stimuli to feel aroused. Ironically, this may be worse than full-blown erectile dysfunction because a man might be less likely to seek help if he can still perform to some extent. Instead of getting to the source of the problem, which could be hormonal decline, men mistakenly search for answers that could be destructive. They begin to blame their mate for not being attractive or attentive enough. They realize a new woman excites them, but they don't put the puzzle together to realize that, with more decline and more familiarity with the new mate, pretty soon, that, too, will not be enough. By then, the levels of hormones decline to the point of putting them in the *no-interest* group, and there's a good chance they'll go down the path of a sexless *second* marriage.

Had these men identified the real problem and remedied their hormonal needs, they may not have had a need to search in all the wrong places. There is even a name for male hormonal decline—*andropause*. Perhaps, if it was understood as well as the female counterpart, menopause, men would take it more seriously.

JOHN'S WANING INTEREST IN SEX

(RF) When I met John, in his mid-nineties and one of the richest men in America, I mentioned that I was a student of aging, and he was kind enough to offer some advice. My ears were wide open and I was happy to hear what he had to say, except when it came to sex. "That's over with," he said. "It just doesn't work anymore at this age."

I told John that's no longer true, and if he was interested, I could bring him to Dr. Morgan and get him back in the saddle. Maybe he thought I meant horseback riding because he said, "That's not going to happen." "No, really," I said. He wasn't interested. How sad.

Somewhere on the road to ninety-four something happened that made this extraordinary fellow give up. He was now in a sexless marriage, and most people would say, "At ninety-four, so what if he is?" What many men don't understand is that there is a way to stay in the game until you die as long as you stay in relatively good health.

This ninety-four-year-old had perfect health except for the changes associated with the expected decline in hormones that affect everyone at some point. John remained sexually active for a long time, but it finally got him when he could no longer achieve an erection, even with the little blue pill. More onerous, however, when I met him he no longer cared, just as Mother Nature intended. But maybe it's time to fool Mother Nature.

The loss of hormone production may not impact both members of a couple at the same time in life—and it may have been this way for John. One or the other mate may experience decline first and lose interest in sex, and the partner may go out and seek sexual partners elsewhere. In John's case, he had a reputation as a ladies' man, so it's possible this happened in his marriage. Some couples who live in sexless marriages find that one, or sometimes both, are still having sex, just not with each other.

John's scenario of losing function and interest in sex is played out rather often, though it usually begins with much younger men. It starts in the forties, occurs more and more in the sixties, and blossoms in the seventies. Remember the statistics: having sex around sixteen times a year by the seventies? Yeah, that could be a problem for some.

Had John entertained replenishing his hormones years before, he would very likely have been able to enjoy sexual activities well into his nineties instead of experiencing the type of decline so common with advancing age. Besides the sexual abilities afforded BHRT, his bones, brain, and body would have aged much better than they had by the time I caught up with him. This didn't have to become the typical story of getting old.

Male Orgasm

There isn't much need to describe or question the existence of the male orgasm. It exists, it feels great, and it gets guys to do stupid things. Enough said. However, there are some interesting facts you might find useful.

- Orgasm and ejaculation are not the same thing. Men can have dry orgasms, though it is not common.

- Men have G spots too: the frenulum (the band of tissue connected to the head of the penis and the shaft) as well as the prostate gland that can be massaged from within the anus pressing toward the front of the body.

- Men typically take less than 7 minutes to reach orgasm, but as most know, this depends on many factors.

- Over the course of a lifetime, a man will release 14 gallons of ejaculate. If men only considered the local sperm bank, they could retire early with that much ejaculate.

- Men have a point of no return called ejaculate inevitability.

- Based on psychological and physical factors, the male orgasm lasts from 5–22 seconds.

Erectile Dysfunction—ED—Impotence

Men experience depression, embarrassment, and a diminished sense of masculinity when they are unable to achieve or maintain an erection. Only about thirty percent of men with erectile dysfunction problems ever seek professional help,[1] which is just plain sad. Going to someone for help usually involves a great deal of courage and desperation. Human sexuality studies teach that most men wish to be the world's greatest lover. Many of them think they are, so when problems arise, they are devastated.

Men with erectile dysfunction (ED) tell me (RM), "that part of me is dead." There is a saying: *fear* is the first time you cannot get it up, *panic* is the second time you cannot get it up. A man feels a responsibility to be a good lover. When he is unable to function the way he feels he should, his sense of masculinity suffers enormously. A man may see himself as no longer being a good provider. A man may think a relationship with a new woman is not possible. How do you disclose this when you're dating, or married?

The Mechanism of Action with Erectile Dysfunction

The blood vessels of the penis are not working properly, either by not supplying enough blood to the chambers in the penis, or by letting the blood leave before it should (hence, the inability to maintain an erection). This blood flow problem may be physical, psychological, or chemical in nature.

Physical ED

The vast majority of men with persistent erectile dysfunction have a physical basis for their problems. The physical changes that account for true erection problems are almost too subtle to detect during a routine physical exam and often require a detailed history and sophisticated tests to confirm ED.

Physical erectile dysfunction means that the plumbing (blood vessels, nerves and/or erectile chambers of the penis) is not in working order. There are many reasons this may happen.

- Clogged arteries (arteriosclerosis) related to heart disease affect almost every artery in your body. If your heart vessels are clogged, so are the vessels leading to your penis.

- Diabetes mellitus also causes physical damage to blood vessels everywhere, including your penis. While many men with diabetes and/or arterial sclerosis can still have great sex, the disease process is ongoing and in time will usually affect their erections, if they don't succumb to heart disease first.

• Men who have experienced a prostatectomy (removal of the prostate gland) or an orchiectomy (removal of testicles) are usually unable to achieve an erection. Often this is because there has been nerve damage (even with the nerve-sparing prostatectomy surgical procedure). Nerves tell the penile blood vessels to relax so the dorsal vein of the penis can engorge with blood and become erect. With nerve damage these signals get disrupted.

• Spinal cord injury is another physical problem that results in ED.

• Obesity, especially excess belly fat, can interfere with sexual function in many ways. It can hinder blood flow to the penis, cause testosterone to plummet, and increase estrogen, which is stored in fat cells.

Psychological ED

Psychogenic impotence is often related to performance anxiety, guilt, embarrassment, and a host of other personal issues. The mind has great power in directing the blood vessels to work for or against the erection. Just think how looking at a naked woman can be enough to arouse a guy, or how someone surprising this same guy in the middle of sex can see the erection disappear.

Chemical ED

Medications, i.e. chemicals, can also have dual effects on erectile function. Some can inhibit sexual response (certain blood pressure medications, antidepressants, and even over-the-counter medications like pseudoephedrine—cold medicine). Other medications can have the opposite effect, as seen in Viagra-type drugs, testosterone, and other hormones, as well as various over-the-counter supplements, such as tribulus, ginseng, ginkgo biloba, and others.

Testing for Erectile Dysfunction

If you wish to discover whether you are capable of getting an erection at all, there is an at-home test you can do. Put a strip of stamps around your flaccid penis when you go to sleep. If you awaken and the stamps are ripped, you had at least one erection during your sleep. This is not the most sophisticated test, but it does help you to know if you are still having erections. If the stamps are stuck to your penis, you probably had a nocturnal emission, too. If you awaken and find a letter in your underpants, your wife has a great sense of humor.If none of your erections are more than 50-percent firm, there is a physical problem and it is important to find the exact cause. For example, it wouldn't be prudent to give you Viagra and find out you had dropped dead in the middle of sexual activity because no medical professional had ever looked into the possibility that your ED was due to clogged arteries.

There is a simple test you can take to learn to what degree you may have ED. It is called the *Sexual Health Inventory for Men (SHIM)* and it is based on your sexual performance over the past six months. It's easy to find this test online and takes less than four minutes to complete.[2] And women can take this test on behalf of their mates because, more than anyone, they already have a good take on their guy's sexual abilities.

Help for Erectile Dysfunction (ED)

Several methods of help for erectile dysfunction (ED) are available.

- Medications—Viagra and various other prescription medications (Viagra was the first to make a big splash on the market and is therefore the best known, but it is just one of several oral medications that can help resolve erectile dysfunction).
- Vacuum pump
- Erection ring
- Intracavernous penile injections
- Penile implants
- Testosterone replacement (*See* Chapter 8)

Treatments for Erectile Dysfunction (ED)—Medications

One in five men in their fifties cannot get a good erection any longer.[3] It's time to do something about this, and the time is now.

Each night, your body tries to achieve several erections that are usually associated with dreams. It's fairly difficult to be anxious when you're asleep, so the sleep test gives the doctor a picture of your physical erection potential. Sexologists do a sophisticated at-home test where they have you place two small rings around your penis before going to sleep to measure frequency and duration of erections. The results are supposed to show four to five erections every night, some lasting forty-five minutes.

Viagra—The Original Blue Pill for ED

Viagra has been shown to *safely* treat erectile dysfunction (ED) in men with the following health conditions: depression, diabetes, heart disease (as long as you are not taking nitrates), and high blood pressure. Try it if you need it. You'll like it.

Viagra was discovered somewhat serendipitously. Viagra (Sildenafil) was a medication that was intended to have a significant effect on clogged arteries. It didn't work so well for all clogged arteries, but men noticed it helped with the blood vessels of their penises. Viagra's maker, Pfizer, really hit the jackpot on this when the first *anti-aging medication,* as they called it, was approved—suddenly Pfizer Pharmaceuticals had a huge hit on their hands.

(RM) I find that many men have low testosterone and require testosterone replacement (*See* Chapter 8). Some even require testosterone replacement and Viagra. Men tell me that, with aging, the strength of their orgasms have gone from a bang to a bust. While in years past, they saw semen explode high in the air, requiring safety goggles for them and their partners, the flow has now been reduced to a dribble, with the thrill of orgasm paralleling this reduction.

Viagra usually does nothing for libido (sexual desire), but it does create a firm erection. This erection then often makes men more excited and confident, which tends to increase the libido.

Viagra works for approximately 70 percent of men.[4] Success is rather good for men with anxiety and other forms of psychogenic impotence, but those with physical problems, (also called plumbing problems) may require other forms of treatment.

Some women become upset when they first discover it is Viagra, and not excitement for them, that is causing his stimulation. But if they understood that Viagra is a medical treatment for an aging warrior, they would not take it personally. Though there is the joke about the guy who calls up his doctor frantically telling him that he took Viagra before leaving work and didn't realize his wife was playing bridge when he returned home. What was he supposed to do with his erection? The doctor suggests that he use his Viagra-induced erection on his maid and the guy replies, "I don't need Viagra when I'm with the maid."

Now, twenty-year-old men take it for fun and eighty-year-old men take it to function. It is popular because it gives older guys their life back. For others, it is recreational in that it allows them to have more sex and better sex than if they just relied on Mother Nature. It is not recommended for, nor is it supposed to be prescribed for, recreational sex. Before you use it in that fashion, recognize that, like all things too good to be true, there may be some yet-to-be-discovered adverse effects of its recreational use besides the known problems (listed below) associated with these types of drugs. You may get so dependent on it that sex without it could seem unsatisfying. If you perform well without medications for erectile dysfunction (ED), you would be wise to avoid them until necessary—plus not all women, even young ones—will find extended sexual intercourse as much of the exciting ride you think it will be.

Viagra doesn't give an instant erection. Physical stimulation is more likely required for those who have true ED, while younger men with either no ED issues or mild problems can still use their imaginations like they used to by thinking about sexual things to allow for the genesis of an erection.

Viagra has been used by a lot of men. It is relatively safe in that, after filling millions of prescriptions, there have not been too many problems other than those that are more common and mild. As long as you understand that everything has some level of risk, you don't have to be afraid to use Viagra.

How to Take Viagra for Maximum Effectiveness

The usual dose is 100 mg; some men do well with 50 mg. Viagra is taken on an empty stomach, which means one hour before or two hours after eating or drinking. It usually remains in your system for six hours.

Viagra Contraindications, Risks, and Side Effects

Here are several important contraindications you should know about.

- Do not take Viagra-type medicines if your doctor prescribed nitrates (nitroglycerin and other similar drugs for your heart) as this may cause a sudden, unsafe drop in your blood pressure.

- Older men, or those with liver or kidney problems, should start on a lower dose of Viagra, 25 mg. Your doctor should be the one who knows all these exceptions and rules. Just make sure you follow his/her instructions. While men often think more is better when it comes to sex, too much Viagra can hurt you.

- All medications have the risk of side effects. Viagra and Viagra-type drugs, in particular, have risks for which you should be cautioned. On the Viagra (Pfizer) website, they have page after page where they discuss the concerns, warnings, contraindications, and adverse reactions.[5]

- Most common side effects are facial flushing (your face turns red and may feel hot), headaches, and upset stomach.

- Less common side effects, mainly affecting vision, include briefly occurring bluish vision, blurred vision, or sensitivity to light. In rare instances, men taking these types of drugs reported a sudden decrease or loss of vision. The website states it is not possible to tell if these events are related directly to the medication or to other factors. You are then warned to stop taking the medication and call a doctor right away. I don't think they needed that warning, because the moment you realized you went blind you were probably going to stop the medicine anyway and call your doctor.

- The site also mentions priapism, the rare event of an erection lasting more than four hours, and says you should seek immediate medical help to avoid long-term injury. It's not enough that you might go blind; you could end up as the target in a game of ring toss.

- The site then notes that a sudden decrease or loss of hearing has been reported (rarely) in people taking Viagra-type medications. They are not sure if this is from Viagra or from other factors. Oh yes, and you should stop the medication and contact your doctor right away.

- Make sure your doctor performs a thorough medical exam to ensure that you are healthy enough to engage in sexual activity. Specifically, they say, "If you experience chest pain, nausea, or any other discomforts during sex, seek immediate medical help."

- The website further warns that Viagra should not be used with other treatments that cause erections. They don't want you to overdose and end up with priapism or a heart attack.

VIAGRA'S PLUSES AND MINUSES

Raymond didn't want to be untrustworthy. He just thought Mary, his new love interest, would be disappointed in him if he stopped using Viagra because then his penis wouldn't be as hard, and he wouldn't be able to have sex as vigorously or as often.

This is very common when men date women years (sometimes decades) younger than them, but it could also happen at any time in a new or established relationship.

Viagra does make a normal erection firmer and reliable, even in new loving encounters, a situation that can cause performance issues for some men like Raymond.[6] This is because sometimes, when a new love discovers her man has been using Viagra, she views it as trust issue. She thought he was so erect because *she* turned him on.

Raymond and Mary were able to work through this issue and went on to develop a loving relationship, with Viagra in the picture.

Other Viagra-like Drug Treatments
for Erectile Dysfunction (ED)

In addition to Viagra, there are about four other oral prescription medications used to treat ED (Cialis, Levitra, Staxyn, Stendra), and basically they all do the same thing—they allow the blood vessels in the penis to dilate in such a manner that blood flows into the penis, resulting in a firm erection. The difference between these medications has primarily to do with *how long each works* and *how long it takes each to work.*

Viagra may be the best-known prescription drug for erectile dysfunction, but Levitra lasts a little longer than Viagra (5 hours versus 4 hours). They both take effect in about thirty minutes. Cialis works faster, in about fifteen minutes, and lasts much longer (up to 36 hours). Staxyn is an orally disintegrating tablet (dissolves under your tongue) that has the same active ingredient as Levitra. Stendra works in around fifteen minutes and lasts around six hours. There is even a low-dose version of Cialis that is taken daily, thus allowing you to be ready all of the time, or so they claim.

You may want to try each brand to see which one works best for you. It is best to get these medications from your doctor for advice and safety issues. While these medications are available on the Internet, without guidance from your doctor and not knowing if the online medication is the real drug, you put yourself at risk.

More Treatments for Erectile Dysfunction (ED)

The Vacuum Pump

There are **vacuum devices** that require using a suction pump to fill the penis with blood followed by placing a rubber ring (erection ring) at the base of the penis to retain the blood while engaging in sex. If pumps were such a great option, you would hear more about them. Some men try them and then stop because they find them ineffective. Some men love the pump. If it works for you, that's great.

There is a big downside if you are trying to be secretive, i.e. if you don't want your partner to know you are using something for ED.

The giveaway is the telltale ring around the base of your penis. It's not easy to explain why you have a rubber ring sitting there. Don't try, "It's my wedding ring," as it won't work.

For couples where the woman is understanding and desirous, this device may be fine.

Erection Ring

As noted, an erection ring is used to retain blood within the penis when using a vacuum pump. It can also be used alone to keep an erection longer in men who don't need the pump to achieve an erection, but could use a little help with maintaining it. These rings are also used recreationally by some men with no ED problems, but rather to enhance the sexual experience. They also go by the name cock ring.

Penile Implants

Penile implants are often inserted at the same time as a prostatectomy (surgical removal of the prostate). They work fairly well. Two hollow chambers are placed within the paired cavities of the penis called the *corpus cavernosa*. A pump is placed within the scrotum. When a man is ready to have sex, he squeezes the scrotal pump repeatedly, which causes water to be transferred to the penile cylinders and creates an erection until the man deflates the implant. To deflate the implant the man squeezes another area so the penis can return to the flaccid state. Patients tell me the implant is good, but not the same. This method works for the more difficult situations, like men with spinal cord injuries. With the implant there can be a valvular problem and the prosthesis has the possibility of springing a leak.

Intracavernous Penile Injections

In 1983, at an annual meeting of the American Urological Association, a maverick British physiologist named Giles Brindley did some urologic theater during his lecture. Dr. Brindley began: "Ladies and Gentleman, thank you for allowing me the opportunity to present to you my lecture today. Approximately 15 minutes ago I injected my right corpus cavernosum (the erectile chambers of the penis) with 30 mg of papaverine (a medicine that dilates the blood vessels, in this case, in the penis)." Then he stepped out from behind the podium, noted that he had no feelings of sexual arousal, dropped his pants, and stood there buck-naked with a full erection. He then walked up and down the aisles so his colleagues could get a better look and make sure he wasn't fooling them with a penile prosthesis. The era of penile injections had arrived.[7]

There was finally an effective treatment for ED.

If you have a penis, you can get an erection thanks to medical science. Penile injections have been in use for over thirty years, but until recently, not too many people knew about them.

While serious side effects are rare, some men can end up with an erection that won't go away if they take too much of the medication. As with Viagra, priapism is an erection lasting more than four hours. This is a medical emergency and is treated in the emergency room, either by surgical intervention, an opposite-acting medication, such as pseudoephedrine, or an injection of terbutaline, whose mechanism of action is unknown. But by taking the prescribed dose your doctor determined is right for you, priapism should not happen. If you decide on your own to increase the dose recklessly, the penis you damage may be your own.

If the injection is used more than three times a week, and the man does not alternate sides where the medication is injected, scar-tissue buildup can occur, which may result in a curved penis when erect. This is called *Peyronie's disease.*

Some men experience a burning discomfort with one of the three medications found in the injection. If this occurs, a prescription with other medications that have less chance of untoward side effects is offered.

Penile injections also gave researchers a way to study erections with an activated penis, without requiring patients to be aroused while they poked and prodded with medical equipment to determine the source of the problem. Penile injections have allowed doctors and researchers to learn how erections work and how they fail.

Men cringe at the thought of putting a needle in their penis until they learn it is easy and almost completely painless. The injection works in minutes no matter whether the stomach is full or empty, unlike Viagra-type medications that should be taken on an empty stomach to achieve erection.

The goal is to have an erection that lasts approximately forty-five minutes. If necessary, this allows the man to please his partner even after he has experienced orgasm.

While injecting the penis to achieve an erection sounds scary, painful, and difficult to accomplish, it's not particularly different from the person with diabetes who has to inject daily to sustain life. The needles are tiny and those who give themselves daily insulin shots say this penile injection is easier. Sure there are differences—an injection in the stomach or arm versus the penis (ouch), and one is lifesaving while the other is for recreational/procreation purposes, which you could argue might be a form of relationship-saving.

Most men who have a libido would define their sexuality as one of the highlights of life. If they can no longer get or maintain an erection, in a manner of speaking this is tantamount to dying. If they tried non-prescription supplements to no avail, if they tried Viagra and failed, if they are very aware of the possibility for the multiple side effects of drugs that affect the entire body and therefore want to avoid drugs, or if health reasons preclude the use of Viagra, the intracavernous injection is the way to go.

With penile injecting, the goal is to get very good at this technique for both pleasure and safety. If you learn to do it right, you will be performing like a porn star. If you don't heed the warnings, you'll be performing like an emergency room patient.

The big risk you want to avoid is priapism. That's the four-hour-plus erection that the Viagra advertisements warn about that everyone thinks would be a dream. It's not. Any erection that is rock hard and lasts for several hours is painful and frightening. Not only is the erection painful after a period of time, but you won't be able to urinate while erect. Since this can cause bladder pain, make sure to empty your bladder before you inject, and try not to drink a gallon of fluids for the hour or so before injecting.

The mere fear of this complication and the fear of injecting could keep many men from trying this most amazing and generally safe method of treating ED. If you do experience priapism, there are some things you can try before heading off to the emergency room. First of all, you don't have to wait four hours to decide to take action. If you are rock hard for more than two hours, you may want to begin taking action. A dose of over-the-counter pseudoephedrine (30 mg repeated every four hours) may help, as will running in place and an icepack applied to the groin. Trying to go to sleep may help. There is a chance you will wake up feeling fine, but if the hours go by with continued pain, this is a medical emergency.

At your initial visit for intracavernous penile injections, the doctor will give you an injection in the office to make sure you respond well, usually starting with a very small dose to see how it works. You may then be told to increase the dose gradually until you achieve the desired result.

Over time, only you, with some experimentation, will be able to determine the perfect dose to achieve the desired erection. You may notice that sometimes the current dose is working better or worse than usual. This means you may have to change the dose from time to time, depending on several factors, including your body chemistry (your hormones can vary from day to day and they do decrease over time), the age of the drug being used (the potency can diminish over time), your psyche (mood and libido may affect the way you respond to these drugs), and probably a host of other variables.

Knowing that your most effective dose may need to be adjusted periodically will help you achieve the desired erection on a consistent basis. However, you must recognize that sometimes it may not work as well, other times it may be too strong, requiring a downward adjustment. Learning to perfect your dose will increase your satisfaction with this method of treating ED. A major caution you must heed is to avoid trying to get a bigger, better erection by increasing the dose too fast. That will get you in trouble and could require an embarrassing emergency room visit.

Because your penis will probably perform better than ever, there is the chance that it may get sore from use. For the first time in years, and possibly the first time ever, you have a very rigid penis that can engage in sex for up to an hour or longer even after orgasm.

One of the recommended features of intracavernous therapy is that you can continue to perform after your orgasm in order to satisfy your partner. Remember, many women are capable of multiple orgasms. Not too many guys have sex for forty-five minutes—three to five minutes is the average—and after that much time of engaging in sex, both partners may find themselves feeling sore.

As much as you might think having sex for an hour would be great, it's probably not. If her orgasm actually takes an hour, remember that utilizing foreplay often helps to even the differences in timing your orgasms. Foreplay often brings more joy and satisfaction to sex as well, so if you are not already engaging in foreplay, both you and your partner may benefit greatly from the pleasure it brings.

The instructions say that you must keep the solution refrigerated at all times, and that it has a shelf life of six months or so. It is sent to you in dry ice to keep it from warming up. If you are going on vacation, you don't need to keep it on ice, you can travel with some loaded syringes that will be effective for a month or longer, even when kept in your luggage, in a hot car, or in your hotel room (though none of this is recommended).

The vial of medication can remain active for well over a year beyond the expiration date, but using outdated medication may result in an infection if the solution becomes contaminated. The medication remains more stable if kept refrigerated as instructed, but the big reason for warning about refrigeration and shelf life is more likely to prevent bacterial growth in the vial that could then cause your penis to become infected. Purchasing your solution from a pristine compounding pharmacy that is careful about sterility helps assure that you don't get contaminated medicine.

One way to help prevent contamination of the solution on your end is to use sterile techniques when loading your needle syringes. Don't touch the needle or the rubber diaphragm on the top of the vial. Use your alcohol gauze to wipe the diaphragm clean before and after loading the needle syringe. Keep your vial of medication in a pill bottle (your pharmacist can get you a pill bottle that will hold it.). Having a capped pill bottle to hold your vial of injectable medication reduces the chance of contamination. An added benefit would be to have your pharmacy provide your prescription in several smaller vials so you can use up the medication in increments. If you purchase 15 ml, ask them to provide you with three 5 ml vials. This way you have a fresh batch of the medication every few weeks, or months, depending on how often you use it.

The basic rules of engagement are as follows.

- Try not to use intracavernous injections more than three times a week.

- Alternate injecting: left side—right side. Do not inject in the same spot too often or you may get scarring inside your penis. Injecting about an inch from the base of your penis at 2 o'clock or 10 o'clock may be most comfortable, since this part of the penis is not getting as much friction as the middle of the penis does during sexual activity.

- Adjust your dose carefully and always try to find the lowest dose that gets the required result. Your dose may change for no apparent reason. One day it may not work well, while another day it seems too strong. Adjust accordingly, and don't let this frighten you.

- If you experience priapism, and it doesn't respond to simple remedies, get to an emergency room.

- Your doctor who prescribes the medication should examine your penis every time you need to renew your prescription to make sure you are not scarring or otherwise causing damage.

The Fine Art of Intracavernous Injections—
Do You Tell Your Partner?

The injections may cause bruise marks on your penis. This is rather common if you don't follow the rule requiring you to press the site of injection with a sterile alcohol gauze pad for at least one full minute—preferably two minutes after the injection. These black and blue (actually purple) marks go away in a matter of two to five days, and they don't hurt. However, try explaining this to your partner if they don't know that you use injections. The best excuse is to tell them that you must have broken a small blood vessel while they were wildly jumping around on your rigid penis. It sounds reasonable. If they don't believe your broken-blood-vessel excuse, they'll think you have some kind of disease, so it's best to follow the rules.

It's even easier if your partner knows you use the injections, but you have to decide whether or not you wish to tell your mate about using them, or, for that matter, even Viagra. Some women may be disappointed and even insulted that you needed an agent to achieve an erection. They don't understand that the problem you are having is not related to them, and they can take it personally unless you explain. If you explain and they are still miffed, or if they ridicule you, then you may want to reconsider having a relationship with someone who lacks compassion or concern for you.

If you decide to avail yourself of these injections, whether or not to tell your partner is the first decision you need to make. If the answer is no, and you're careful and plan accordingly, it's not difficult to use these injections undercover (not to be read *under the covers*). Most people understand that you may want to use the bathroom before engaging in sex. You have your needle preloaded and hidden under your sink, ready to use at the time you excused yourself to go to the bathroom. For the times you are away from home, you can find ways to carry the syringe on your person. The only time a big difficulty may arise is in a spontaneous situation where you may still be able to excuse yourself to go to the bathroom in the middle of petting. Don't expect to tear off her dress, pull her to the floor, and engage in lustful sex. That ain't happening in your world unless you use Viagra and time it right. That's a scene for the movies anyway.

Overall, it is best to be forthright with your mate and let her know you use this medication to have sex, but maybe it would be better not to let her know on the first encounter. Once someone falls for you, thinks you are amazing in bed, or at least likes you, they may be much more sympathetic and accepting than if they were to learn about your problem before they get to know you.

An elderly gentleman courted this sexually sophisticated woman, and she played hard to get for several dates. When she finally decided to sleep with this fellow, he told her all about his need to inject his penis, and went off to get himself ready. The admission and description of the process completely freaked out the woman who beat a hasty retreat from his apartment while he was injecting. Poor guy came out to his empty apartment with a fully erect penis and nothing to do with it.

Premature Ejaculation—PE

Ejaculation has to do with nerves and muscular contractions that are controlled by physical contact and that are, especially, under the control of the mind, which can have an enormous effect on all aspects of sexual response. One form of premature ejaculation is when the man becomes so excited that he cannot control himself and ejaculates *before* his penis becomes rigid. The reason for this is that ejaculation has a separate set of controls from erection and can take place even when the penile blood vessels don't fill to the top.

Premature ejaculation (PE) affects a man's self-esteem, and his sense of sexuality and attractiveness. PE is described as achieving climax either before penetration or shortly thereafter. It's not difficult to imagine how PE can interfere with a man's willingness to enter into loving and intimate relations.

(RM) When asking my male patients how long they think the average sexual encounter lasts after penetration, they often respond "about 15–20 minutes." Really? It occurs to me that they may be including the begging and the foreplay in their estimates. Twenty minutes? They may be counting cocktails and snacks in their calculations because one sexual study, for example, showed that the median time from vaginal penetration to ejaculation in humans is 5.4 minutes.[8] Fifty members of the Society for Sex Therapy research (all professionals) did a survey study and they found that *adequate* sex lasted from 3–7 minutes; *desirable* sex lasted from 7–13 minutes; *too short* was from 1–2 minutes; and *too long* was from 10–30 minutes.[9]

Some odd PE cures, such as thinking about death, are reported in the medical literature. Why get started having sex if you're going to think about old Aunt Matilda, rest her soul? Other solutions suggest biting the inside of the cheek to cause pain, thinking about sports, masturbation before sex with their partners so it will take longer to climax the second time (this may also require planning, as much added time may be needed before a new erection can materialize), using one or more condoms to decrease sensation, using creams to anesthetize the penis, and antidepressants that inhibit a climax. Before going onto medications, you might want to try any of these easy methods.

Treatments for Premature Ejaculation (PE)

Viagra has no effect on ejaculation, but for some, premature ejaculation is best treated by using it or other ED medications, or having intracavernous penile injections. By feeling secure about maintaining the erection, some men are less likely to release early, especially if the PE is related to fear of erectile dysfunction. Even if they do, their recovery time is usually faster. And the second time around, they will often last much longer to satisfy even the most difficult partner. With this enhanced confidence, the PE fades in time.

If three minutes of stimulating sexual activity can be deemed adequate, what is premature? Too much less than adequate puts you into the PE category. For some men, ten to thirty seconds is PE and certainly not much time to please a partner, unless foreplay is employed. For other couples, however, given the proper amount of foreplay, ten seconds of frenzy might be sufficient to feel satisfied.

Before Viagra and intracavernous injections, the classic treatment for premature ejaculation was the *choke technique* of the penis. To understand how this treatment works, you need to understand that a few moments before the man's orgasm there is a point after which he cannot hold back—even if there is no more direct stimulation of any kind.

The challenge is for the man to be able to identify when he is nearing the point of no return without crossing over the line. If he can do this, in theory anyway, he can stop physical stimulation and defer ejaculation. If the penis is squeezed firmly, *choked,* at this moment, it further helps to halt ejaculation. This takes a lot of practice to become effective. For some it doesn't work, or it seems like more work than it's worth—when a man is about to ejaculate, he really has little interest in choking his penis to stop the process.

Since much PE is related to psychological issues, this method may prove to be disappointing. Some men who experience PE can actually have an orgasm without any stimulation, which means that even if they are not engaged in thrusting, they would still reach orgasm.

One of the more effective treatments for PE has been the use of SSRIs—a special class of antidepressants. As an unexpected side effect, these medications can delay ejaculation in some men. Some of these medications are to be taken only when men are about to have sex, while others require small doses every day.

Male-Enhancement Supplements for Treatment of PE (also ED)

As an alternative to all the prescription remedies, it may be best to first try some supplements to see if they can help your PE and ED. After all, a noble prize was awarded to three researchers for their discoveries concerning how nitric oxide helps signal blood flow.[10] The amino acid *arginine* is the only nutrient that essentially produces nitric oxide in the body. Enhancing nitric oxide may help erectile dysfunction by getting more blood flow to the penis. This benefit is even noted on the website for the National Institutes of Health.[11] Using this knowledge, many supplements have come to market to enhance this process.[12] The most common remedies that seem to be effective for ED and PE include: acetyl L carnitine, L-arginine, alpha ketoglutarate, Asian ginseng, deer antler velvet, ginkgo biloba, muira puama, and tribulus terrestris.

Brands may come and go, but some of the brand names that contain various levels of these ingredients include Agri-Vive III, Ultra Turbo, and Ultimate Vigor from Real Advantage Nutrients, Primal Max from Primal Force, and Jonathan Wright's Male Formula and his Vicariin Virility Formula as distributed by Tahoma Clinic Dispensary. You should do some research to find a product that has good ingredients and a better reputation. (See Resources in back.)

Most of these remedies make claims of providing stronger, harder erections allowing you to *go all night*. You may wish to avoid this hype, but since some men find these remedies effective, you may find that they can work for you, too. If you do want to try them, show the ingredients to your medical doctor or pharmacist and do detailed research to make sure the ingredients will not make you ill. If the company doesn't list every ingredient, avoid them. Some of the side effects of remedies containing other ingredients than those noted above include rapid heart rate, anxiety, and an overall antsy feeling.

Try to make your purchases from a company that offers a money-back guarantee so if the product doesn't work for you, you can get your money back. The more reputable companies are more likely to test their formulas for quality and concentration.

Exercises for PE, ED, and Incontinence

Kegel exercises may be something men should consider as part of their program to manage ED and PE, as well as issues with incontinence. While these exercises have been used by women for years to manage incontinence, researchers are now studying Kegel benefits for men.

For men, the exercise requires tightening the muscles used to cut off the flow of urine. Each contraction is held for a few seconds, then released. Repeat 10–15 times each day if your doctor feels it's alright in your situation.

Definitive results are not yet in, but Dr. Andrew Spiegel, a urologist, describes Kegel exercises as benefiting men in many ways.[13]

The Prostate Gland and Its Many Issues

No discussion of male sexuality is complete without an examination of the prostate's role in it. First thing, what exactly is the prostate? The healthy prostate is the size of a walnut; it is right under the bladder and within the rectum, and it surrounds the urethra. Muscles in the prostate help move sperm and they also help open the bladder so urine can pass through the prostate. This is when the prostate is normal, but if the prostate is enlarged and puffy, which in doctor talk is BPH (benign prostatic hypertrophy), the passage of urine can be blocked. For optimal urinary and sexual function, it is necessary to have a healthy prostate.

A short history of the prostate gland is useful to an understanding of its importance. Only men have a prostate gland. (Prostate is spelled with one R—it is not prostrate, which means to lay flat.) The prostate increases in size four times in life—at birth, puberty, young adulthood, and around age fifty. Note that these growth spurts all coincide with major hormonal changes. The prostate produces male hormones, along with the adrenal glands and the testicles.

The prostate gland rarely troubles men before the age of fifty. But, as noted, over a lifetime, it does gets bigger, resulting in BPH—benign prostatic hypertrophy. This is a very common condition—nearly 90 percent of men after fifty are affected to some degree. BPH tends to get worse with age and this causes men to wake up several times during the night to urinate, a sleep disruption that leads to low energy and fatigue. BPH can affect sexual performance that, in turn, may result in mood changes, erectile dysfunction (ED), depression, anxiety, and even the sexless marriage.

Symptoms of Benign Prostatic Hypertrophy

Men with BPH will experience some or all of the following symptoms:

- Awakening at night to urinate, maybe even every two hours
- Decreased force of urination
- Difficulty starting your stream of urine
- Feelings of incomplete emptying
- Increased frequency of urination
- Painful urination
- Reduced flow
- Urgency to urinate immediately
- Urinary blockage (go to the Emergency Room)
- Urinary leakage—dripping

The PSA Test

Prostate specific antigen, a protein made by the prostate gland, is given off in higher amounts by enlarging (as in BPH) and/or cancerous prostate glands. Measuring this protein is the basis of the PSA test which has been credited with detecting 70 percent of all prostate cancers. Prostate cancer is very slow growing and is one of the most curable cancers.

No need to be frightened if your PSA score is high, since many cases of increased PSA indicate BPH or prostatitis (inflammation of the prostate). A high PSA merely indicates the need for a workup to rule out prostate cancer.

The PSA, like many laboratory tests, is not a perfect gauge as some men with cancer can have normal PSA levels. Most men with mild or moderately elevated PSA levels do not have cancer. Studies have been done showing that only 25 percent of the men who had biopsies based on an elevated PSA turned out to have prostate cancer.[14]

The Value of PSA Testing and Digital Rectal Examinations

There is currently some controversy over the value of the PSA test versus the number of unnecessary biopsies that have been done based on PSA results. In 2013, The American Urological Association (AUA) recommended that men between the ages of fifty-five and sixty-nine, and men at high risk, discuss the possible benefits and risks of the PSA with their doctors before agreeing to the test and recommended that it not be performed routinely on all men.[15]

Consider having a digital rectal exam. Your doctor will insert a finger about two inches into your rectum and press on the prostate gland. He/she feels for consistency, texture, and size of the gland that may indicate pathology. The exam is uncomfortable, but not painful. Many men avoid this important exam because of embarrassment or fear of pain.

Work with someone well qualified (and with thin fingers) who will look at the entire picture and refer you to a urologist where panoramic integrative medicine is truly being practiced.

Prostate Cancer

The incidence of prostate cancer is rising, but most cases of this cancer are so slow-growing that the majority of men die of something else before the cancer gets them. Prostate cancer is only fatal in aggressive cases. The treatment is often debilitating when it results in ED (erectile dysfunction) and/or incontinence.

The incidence of prostate problems is so high with advancing age that *prevention* is the best way to avoid the consequences. A healthy diet and supplementation are ways to keep ahead of the statistics that predict that most men will likely suffer from some level of prostate involvement.

Other Prostate Issues

As you know, most women *seem* to lose all their hormones over the course of a few months or more (aka menopause). But, men lose their hormones over decades. Between the ages of twenty-five (yes, twenty-five) and fifty, a man's testosterone level decreases by about 50 percent and his estrogen levels increase by 50 percent.[16]

This happens because older men produce more aromatase and that combines with their testosterone to produce more estrogen.

Men go through andropause just the way women go through menopause. Although men's loss of hormones is more gradual, when the increased estrogen is factored in, the effects can be profound and can result in a loss of strength and energy, mood issues, conversion of muscle to fat, memory loss, heart problems (there are testosterone receptors on all your heart cells), [17] increased belly fat, breast enlargement, and loss of sexual energy. This imbalance of testosterone and estrogen ratios accompanies the onset of prostate problems.

Eugene Shippen, M.D., author of *The Testosterone Syndrome*,[18] describes a cascade of events: When men's testosterone levels go down, they gain weight. This increased weight increases estrogen levels even more—the estrogen increases sex hormone-binding globulin (SHBG), which binds testosterone. Now with less active, unbound testosterone there is more weight gain, and then estrogen increases even more. You see the problematic cycle of events.

Speaking of weight gain and diet, knowledge of portions and what a healthy diet entails are of paramount importance. They, too, play a major role in the cycles of life. Various nutrients and minerals all work together. For example, zinc prevents testosterone from converting into estrogen. Less estrogen means less belly fat.

Diet for a Healthy Prostate

By maintaining a healthy diet, you can avoid many problems in your life in general and with your sex life in particular. Don't wait until a problem develops. A few simple changes in your eating habits can reap huge benefits.

- You need protein and even saturated fats (animal fat) to make hormones (testosterone in particular). At all cost, try to buy organic beef and chicken so you are not ingesting synthetic hormones, antibiotics, herbicides, pesticides, and GMO-based corn and wheat (known to be carcinogenic) used as feed.

- Avoid or limit your intake of processed meats (hot dogs, lunch meats, sausages, and others). Cooking meat at high temperatures (as in grilling and broiling) produces heterocyclic amines (HCAs) that may be associated with an increased risk of prostate cancer.

- Eating large amounts of dairy products may increase cell growth in the prostate gland which can lead to cancer.[19] Limit your dairy consumption, but not to exclusion. You need whole fat because it contains CLA (conjugated linoleic acid). CLA enhances metabolism and the feeling of fullness and is anti-carcinogenic. Buy only organic dairy products because you don't want the hormones and other toxic substances found in regular dairy products. What are described as heart-healthy, fat-free, and low-fat products do not have healthy CLAs.

The reason for the association between dairy products and prostate cancer is cow's milk. It may contain large amounts of estrogen, especially today, when dairy farms milk their cows throughout pregnancy, a practice never considered in traditional herding societies. Pregnant cows have much more estrogen in their blood and that means *so do you* if you drink large quantities of milk. To make matters worse, dairy cows are fed synthetic estrogen to fatten them.

- Eat more fish to get the omega-3 fatty acids that have been associated with less prostate cancer risk. Consider supplementing with a high-quality omega-3.

- Eat plenty of cruciferous vegetables (broccoli, Brussels sprouts, cabbage, kale) as they contain a substance that converts into DIM (diindolylmethane) known for its anticancer properties. DIM inhibits prostate cell growth.[20]

- Alcohol consumption should be limited since alcohol decreases the production of all of your hormones. You don't have to be a teetotaler, but daily consumption, especially to excess, does not help your prostate gland or your general health over time. Take a break from daily consumption to let your body reset.

- Soy has weak estrogenic activity. There is controversy as to whether soy causes unhealthy hormonal effects on both men and women. Until this controversy plays out, it is prudent to avoid excessive amounts of soy in any form other than fermented, which seems to be healthy rather than harmful.

- There are prostate-healthy substances you can introduce into your diet for a healthy prostate gland. These include:
  - Selenium—found in Brazil nuts—eat three a day;
  - Pomegranate juice—contains strong antioxidants—drink 4 ounces a day;
  - Lycopene—found in watermelon, papayas, and especially tomatoes—because lycopene is tightly bound in tomatoes, you get more of it when tomatoes are cooked or pureed, or from tomato juice, spaghetti sauce, and even ketchup;

- Green tea contains compounds that appear to be beneficial—drink five cups a day.

Supplementing for Prostate Problems

Because prostate gland problems are a medical problem, it is best to consult with your doctor at the first sign of symptoms. If you wish to try some supplements to see if you can control your problem before going on prescription medication, that is all right, as long as you first rule out prostate cancer by seeing your doctor and telling him/her what supplements you would like to try.

Beneficial supplements for the prostate:

- Saw palmetto. This is the supplement most commonly mentioned for prostate health. It blocks some of the conversion of testosterone to dihydrotestosterone (DHT), a stronger form of testosterone. While DHT *is* needed, if it is too high, hair loss and an enlarged prostate are usually the result. Saw palmetto can be useful here by helping to prevent prostate enlargement.

- Other beneficial supplements include: Beta-sitosterol (enhances saw palmetto), lycopene, pumpkin seeds, pomegranate and beet juice, pygeum extract, quercitin, selenium, vitamin D, vitamin E, and zinc.

Many scientific studies, including those done at the National Institutes of Health (NIH), leading hospitals, and universities, have shown various supplements to be effective in treating infection, pain, prostate enlargement, prostatitis, and urinary matters, in addition to helping prevent prostate cancer.[21,22,23]

Since prostate problems are so common as men age, it may be wise to consider a healthy lifestyle and supplements before you ever have symptoms. Even men in their forties may benefit from prevention. By keeping your prostate healthy, you have a much better chance of keeping your marriage healthy.

There are a good number of supplement companies with integrity out there and it is important to use these reliable companies when you buy supplements. A problem can arise with supplements if the quality and quantity of the self-monitored ingredients is not adequate, thereby making the effectiveness sometimes questionable.

You often get what you pay for in life—the cheapest supplements may not have the best ingredients, and the most costly may be over-priced. Try to find a balanced product from a reliable company. You may consider consulting with a naturopathic practitioner, or you can ask your doctor for an opinion. If they are an integrative physician, they are likely versed on supplements. Do realize that, based on their bias, standard establishment doctors may be more inclined to recommend prescription medications. With medical insurance, the prescription medication may cost less than the supplement, though taking a natural supplement and changing your lifestyle may be the smarter option.

In trying to research the best supplements on the Internet, you should be careful. Some sites appear to be independent guides, but they often rate the most popular products, ones that are usually effective based on their repeat sales to satisfied customers. In their summation, there is always one that they recommend as the *best of the best* while giving applause to several of the well-known products. It truly seems to be an independent analysis, but upon further research, you may find that these sites are really affiliated with the one product they rated the best, thus directing you to their product. If this is the case, their analysis is anything but independent and they may be touting expensive, inferior, and ineffective products.

The best option is to seek out a knowledgeable alternative practitioner for advice or, if you live near a reliable health food store, ask the proprietor what supplements are found to be the most effective—*not* the most sold.

A DECLINING SEX DRIVE

(RM) When I saw Tom, he couldn't actually tell me how often he had sex with his wife. But he was able to tell me they did try to have sex on their wedding anniversary, birthdays, and some holidays. Eventually, Tom told me he didn't really even have sexual feelings or fantasies anymore. He used to enjoy seeing, not touching, beautiful women. Tom thought this must be what happens when you get older. He used to need sex, not just want sex. If his marriage had been this sexless in the past, he might have needed to seek comfort elsewhere. However, after employing some of the methods recommended in this book, Tom's marital sex life picked up, to the delight of both him and his wife.

Prostate Medication

There are several medications prescribed for BPH. They include Avodart, Flomax, Hytrin, Proscar, and others. Even Cialis, the ED medication, has been shown to help. If you can't get the problem under control naturally, the choice of which medication, or combination thereof, is left to your physician.

Propecia (finasteride) is the common prescription used by men to block DHT conversion that helps prevent male-pattern hair loss. Make sure you learn about, and understand, the risks before taking this, or any, prescription medications for hair loss. Propecia is the same medication as Proscar, which is the brand used for BPH. The hair-loss-prevention dose is 1 mg (Propecia) while the BPH dose is 5 mg (Proscar). Don't think you can substitute one for the other.

Learn to be a Good—strike that—Great Lover

So guys, you finally have a workable erection and are ready to get back in the bedroom. Here is some advice for your consideration.

Be patient and build anticipation. Your woman is like an iron. She needs time to warm up before she gets hot enough to take the wrinkles out of your penis. Of course, since you probably don't iron your own clothes, you have no clue, and that's why you are here. Make sure your nails are trimmed (poorly trimmed and jagged nails hurt). It is important to avoid going too fast by heading straight for her clitoris or by fully inserting two fingers. Make sure she is well lubricated, either naturally or with the help of personal lubricants you can purchase at any pharmacy.

Most women reach orgasm by stimulating the clitoris, not by penetration. The clitoris is the small pink button between her inner lips (we are not talking the lips of her mouth). In the beginning, soft rubbing on the supersensitive areas is more appreciated than rough, intense manipulation. Use your middle finger to draw small circles on the inner lips and stop just beneath the clitoris. If this excites her, you can gently touch the clitoris, increasing pressure if she likes it. Your partner will let you know that she is getting excited by making sounds, moving towards your touch, becoming more lubricated, and breathing more heavily.

Starting at the clitoris, you can visualize a clock, with 12 o'clock being the top of the clitoris and 6 o'clock being the vaginal opening.

Explore every hour and learn the places she enjoys the best. Don't be afraid to ask. While men usually prefer to be handled fast and hard, most women prefer to be handled slowly and with a gentle touch until approaching climax at which time you can be more physical.

The G spot is more an area than a spot. Insert your index finger into the vagina to the second knuckle and press upward toward her belly button. Again, go slowly at first, gradually increasing pressure as your partner lets you know she is more excited. Simultaneously providing light pressure around the clitoris enhances her desire.

Oral sex (fellatio and cunnilingus) can be a pleasurable way to engage in sex. Older folks may have little or no experience with this as it was not as common thirty to forty years ago. There is a reason for this lack of practice—prior to 1962, sodomy was actually a felony in every state, punishable by prison and hard labor. Interestingly, in 1779 America, sodomy was punishable by death. By 1986, the Supreme Court was upholding the constitutionality of the sodomy laws, and by 2003 they had reversed their decision that invalidated sodomy in the remaining fourteen states that hadn't already rescinded their sodomy laws. As of April 2014, seventeen states have not yet formally repealed their sodomy laws though they are not actively enforced. Considering this history and the fact that some people are not interested in engaging in oral sex, you may have a reluctant partner. That is, of course, a personal issue with which you have to deal. If both parties have never engaged, but are willing to try, they may find that it enhances their sexual union.

There are many ways that women become stimulated. Besides the physical ways that have such a strong influence on men, women can become more stimulated after they listen to your thoughts and dreams, see how you dress, and feel your full attention when you converse. If you actually ask questions with true curiosity, she will often respond sexually. Women need to talk before sex. They need to connect on an emotional level. If you believe in planning ahead, after engaging in sex, hold your woman in your arms and curl up. This enhances that emotional bond, and if she enjoys the entire process, it's more likely she will enthusiastically participate and even initiate sex.

8

Testosterone

~

It's What Makes a Man a Man

SEXUAL *INTEREST* FOR A BOY BECOMES PROFOUNDLY IMPORTANT once he discovers how good it feels to play with his penis. He doesn't yet know how much power this protruding body part has or how much trouble it can cause. Sexual *desire* begins as a result of the production of the hormone testosterone and intensifies as levels rise during puberty.

A three-year-old boy isn't all that interested in sex, pretty much like most frail ninety-three-year-old men. What they have in common, besides possibly wetting their beds, is that both are running on fumes of testosterone, the hormone that makes them sexual creatures.

In the humblest manner, sex can be described as a hormone-based phenomenon. Hormones put you to sleep at night and wake you in the morning. They control your blood pressure, build and maintain muscle tone, and lubricate joints. Hormones help balance blood sugar, enhance immunity, and resist allergies and infections. They help the body produce energy and burn fat. They fight stress, prevent fatigue, calm anxiety, stabilize mood, and relieve depression. Hormones perform countless functions and provide abundant benefits.

Sexuality begins with hormones and the effect they have on the mind (libido—arousal and sexual desire) and body (development of sexual characteristics such as a deep voice, body hair, quality of the erection, and the production of sperm).

101

While testosterone (T) is the major hormone that changes a boy to a man, many other hormones are involved. The human body has more than fifty different types of hormones besides the common ones everyone hears about, such as testosterone, estrogen, and progesterone.[1]

Hormones are released into the bloodstream every day and control all sorts of critical functions that allow life to happen. The production of nearly every hormone decreases with aging, and as a result of this decline, many functions of the human body become diminished over time.

The first thought most people have about testosterone is that it enhances libido and sexual function, and this is true. Erectile dysfunction medications (Viagra) may enhance the ability to achieve and maintain an erection, but you need to have optimal levels of testosterone to *want* to achieve and maintain an erection.

Low T—Recently Identified as a Problem

New ways of diagnosing, testing, and treating men are often met with resistance and can take decades to happen. Innovative thinking is not often met with open minds and must survive three stages.

1. First, there is rejection;

2. This is followed by ridicule;

3. Then there is an abundance of medical studies stating they always knew this new idea was valid—hence, acceptance.

Suddenly after years of rejection, pharmaceutical companies are advertising that men may be suffering from low T (the term coined by pharmaceutical companies to indicate low testosterone). While just a few years ago, you'd be hard pressed to find any doctors willing to prescribe testosterone, now they do. There is even an online test for men to find out if they have low T so they can then go to their doctors for a prescription.

Symptoms of Low Testosterone

How do you know if you are suffering from low T? How do you know if a testosterone deficiency is contributing to your sexless marriage?

Many times the diagnosis can be suspected if you have a number of the symptoms below that are associated with low T.

- Aches and pains
- Anger
- Anxiety
- Belly fat
- Cold hands and feet
- Decreased sexual performance
- Depression
- Difficulty concentrating
- Diminished quality and duration of erections
- Excessive sweating
- Feeling fatter
- Gaining weight, especially in the gut
- Irritability
- Itching
- Less energy; muscle weakness
- Low sex drive
- Loss of morning and nighttime erections
- Loss of muscle mass
- Loss of self-confidence and self-image
- Love handles
- Man boobs
- Memory problems
- Mood swings
- Morning stiffness (and not the good kind, either)
- Plaque-related heart and circulation problems
- Poor quality sleep
- Reduced sexual arousal
- Slow healing
- Slow recovery from exercise or physical activity
- Thinning bones
- Tired all the time

Causes of Low Testosterone

- Aging is the most common cause of low testosterone and eventually affects everyone
- Addiction, opioid use, and taking certain medications like statins
- Alcohol consumption
- Anabolic steroids

- Anticholinergics (Benadryl, Cogentin, Donnatal, Pro-Banthine)
- Antidepressants (MAO inhibitors, SSRIs, and tricyclics)
- Antifungal medications
- Antihypertensive drugs (Clonadine, Inderal, Lasix, and reserpine)
- Intense exercise
- Marijuana use
- Obesity
- Prednisone
- Tagamet
- Tranquilizers (Haldol, Seroquel, Thorazine, Zyprexa)

Other causes include:

- Deficiencies of vitamin C and zinc increase the conversion of testosterone to estrogen, which is a double whammy—low T and too much estrogen.

- Head trauma. Any head trauma can lower testosterone.[2] Professional athletes in their twenties who experienced head injuries may have low testosterone levels when tested correctly. Although a discussion of how traumatic brain injury may affect hormonal levels, hence mental and physical health, is beyond the scope of this book, just know that even minor bruising to a part of the brain called the anterior pituitary may profoundly reduce the testosterone levels to that of an octogenarian. Imagine a ten-million-dollar contract being given to an athlete with undisclosed octogenarian levels of male hormones (androgens).

- High levels of SHBG. Your body makes sex-hormone-binding globulin. It keeps your testosterone from being used as it is bound to this protein. If SHBG is high, your free testosterone will be lower.

- Testosterone abuse. Ironically, stopping the use of testosterone after abusing it causes low testosterone. Long-term abuse causes men to lose the ability to make their own and requires them to take testosterone for life.

What Happens to Relationships With Untreated Low T?

This condition of low T is not the way you have to live. There is something you can do about improving the quality of your life—or you can believe the present medical wisdom that it is *normal* to be less interested in sex as you age.

To review, testosterone turns a boy into a man and the lack thereof turns a man into an old man. This old man exhibits what is known by European physicians and others as frailty syndrome.[3]

It's easy to diagnose. Just pat this guy on the back or shoulder and if you feel bones and no muscle, he's got this syndrome. Do you really want to age in this manner?

With a progressive decline in testosterone, both the libido/desire and the performance, as defined by the frequency and quality of erection, are diminished. This combination of a lesser libido and lesser erections can easily lead to performance anxiety that often leads to psychological ED, physical ED, or both. Is there any question that these events may result in the sexless marriage that is not improved by conventional marital counseling?

The Required Testing for Low Testosterone

So how does a man know if he has a deficiency or insufficiency of testosterone other than experiencing the many symptoms of a deficiency? By having laboratory tests done. These are crucial.

For Male Hormones

- Total testosterone—not the whole picture
- Free testosterone—the testosterone available for your body to use

For Female Hormones

- Progesterone—if progesterone is low, testosterone converts to estrogen
- Estradiol—if this form of estrogen is high, testosterone can convert into more estrogen
- Estrone—the estrogen found in fat

- Thyroid hormones—TSH, T3, T4 free T3, free T4, TBG, reverse T3, antithyroperoxidase Abs, antithyroglobulin Abs

Other tests that are required to help fill in the picture include:

- Androstenediol
- Androstenedione
- Chemistry profile 14
- Complete blood count (CBC)
- DHEA-S—Dehydroepiandosterone sulfate
- Fasting insulin—receptors for insulin become resistant with aging and overeating
- 5-DHT—5-dihydrotestosterone, a stronger testosterone-like drug, but it can convert into a safer androstenediol
- FSH, LH—indicators of hypothalamus–brain–function
- HCG (Human chorionic gonadotropin)—helps prime your hypothalamus to produce testosterone, and lose weight
- HgbA1C—indicates what your blood sugar has averaged over three months
- HGH. (Human growth hormone)—also known as IGF-1 or somatocedin C
- Homocysteine
- HsCRP
- Lipid profile with VAP
- Liver function tests with GGT
- Prolactin—if high, this is a major cause of erectile dysfunction and loss of libido
- PSA and percent-free PSA (prostate tests)
- Red blood count (RBC)

- SHBG (sex-hormone-binding globulin)—if high, it binds your testosterone, keeping it from being used

- Vitamin C and zinc levels—if low, testosterone converts to estrogen

Why All the Tests?

Taking testosterone is more complicated than just measuring how much you take. One of the very bad consequences of taking testosterone, as noted by the tests described above, is that it can turn into estrogen, the female hormone. And while men need a *little* estrogen, when there is too much, it becomes unhealthy and actually dangerous. This is why testing for estrogen and other female hormones in men is so important.

Low testosterone makes men more prone to many diseases, including Alzheimer's disease and other types of dementia, chronic fatigue, diabetes, heart disease, osteoporosis, and premature death.[4]

How many of these symptoms describe your life? While you could have many of them and not have a testosterone deficiency, if you have several of them, it is time to be examined by a doctor versed in hormone replacement.

It could be argued that these symptoms are merely a description of normal aging. It is normal to lose the ability to produce hormones as you age, and these symptoms will, in time, affect most men to some degree or other. Is this the type of normal aging you want to experience?

With knowledge of the many effects of decreased testosterone, it is perfectly understandable that this change is responsible for many older men no longer looking for excitement in the bedroom. They may also have lost their edge in business affairs, and physical activity may be relegated to leisure walks and watching others engage in sports on television.

Because diminished libido and erectile dysfunction manifest slowly, occurring over many years, the man and his relationship with his wife goes downhill without a clear understanding of the cause. Many women become frustrated and blame themselves or their husbands for their sexless marriage. Those women, who also experience an equal loss of libido, may assume this is the normal state of an aging marriage. This is how many relationships become sexless and feel hopeless. Just maybe it's time to see a doctor to find out for sure if low T is affecting you and your marriage.

If your testosterone has been tested and interpreted correctly, a deficiency is often found. Simply getting a total testosterone level is not enough; other tests are necessary to make a customized treatment program.

All these tests can seem confusing. Do you have to understand them all? No, but your doctor should. Are all these tests really necessary? Most certainly. If you don't know when something is out of balance, your body could be making too much or too little of the hormones that are meant to keep you healthy, as well as producing too much of those that are unhealthy. For all these reasons, it should be evident that taking testosterone requires detailed, appropriate, and routine testing, as well as continued monitoring by someone who is medically knowledgeable about prescribing bio-identical hormones. Many conventional physicians reject hormone replacement and some of the tests described, most probably because they're not trained in the complexities of hormone actions and interactions and appropriate therapy. Taking testosterone from some unknown or unknowledgeable source can be dangerous to your well-being.

Regarding the bio-identical issue as it relates to testosterone, there needs to be some better understanding. Testosterone is testosterone. The actual molecule is bio-identically the same as that produced within your body. The problem arises, not with testosterone itself, but when synthetic methyl or hydroxyl molecules are added to testosterone.

Such drugs as nandrolone and methyltestosterone are the bad players. These synthetic versions of testosterone may become problematic when the body cannot clear them well. They are abused by athletes and are known to cause erectile dysfunction and cardiovascular damage.

There are various topical formulations (Androgel, Testim and others) that are bio-identical testosterone in an alcoholic gel. The problems with these topical gels are mainly related to the alcohol content, the large amount of gel required and its irritability on the skin, plus the unreliability of the dosing. Gels and creams must be applied daily.

Testosterone cypionate and testosterone enanthonate are acid esters of bio-identical testosterone that are injected. The body has to cleave these esters to facilitate allowing the testosterone into the bloodstream. Since this is a slow process, this formulation lasts longer between dosing and injections are not needed daily.

Possibly the most important takeaway message regarding bio-identical testosterone therapy is that it can be safe and effective if it is administered in proper dosing and monitored regularly to make sure the dose remains appropriate and it doesn't convert to dangerous levels of other hormones.

Treatment after Testing

Testosterone isn't just for sex anymore. Yes, it does increase the libido in men and women, but it does much more and the testing helps to determine how it's doing on all fronts.

You have testosterone receptors from your brain to your toes and, like all hormones there are many things it does in the body. (The *many* mechanisms of action also apply to androstenedione, DHEA, dihydrotestosterone, estradiol, estrogen, estrone, human growth hormone (HGH), and progesterone, among others.)

Studies show that testosterone strengthens the heart, lowers LDL and total cholesterol, improves every cardiac risk factor, and promotes healthy blood pressure as well as increases muscle mass.[5]

Testosterone affects so many aspects of your health that not maintaining appropriate levels is pretty much a guarantee of the decline that too many in the conventional medical community consider normal aging. Is it normal to have high blood pressure, high blood sugar, or high cholesterol as you age? Of course it's not. Those are called dysfunctional diseases, often brought about by poor lifestyle choices. Medications are available for these ailments and are readily prescribed. As a result, lives are saved and the quality of life is greatly increased—as, of course, are the risks from taking a voluminous quantity of pills every day. Yet, when it comes to a natural decline in a hormone that affects a host of health and quality-of-life issues, this is referred to as normal aging, even though the remedies for these conditions are at hand and have been for many years.

With so many men experiencing a decline in advancing age, it is surprising how few get treatment. The most likely reasons are because too many doctors are fearful of prescribing testosterone, and most health insurance does not pay for this treatment anyway.

Gels available from your mainstream doctor are often sticky and uncomfortable, and can cause skin irritation or blisters. If you are working with an integrative physician (M.D. or D.O.), they may prescribe compounded testosterone gels that are more concentrated, therefore requiring very small amounts, or periodic injections of the hormone into your buttocks. Gels and injections bypass the necessity for liver detoxification. Compounded hormones are made by pharmacists who specialize in making bio-identical hormones in individualized doses.

Your integrative doctor will do all of the testing, and determine a proper starting dose of testosterone. He/she will test your blood again in a few weeks to see how your levels of testosterone and estrogen are balancing out. Treatment continues as long as you like and as long as there are no adverse consequences—but be mindful that it is the conversion of testosterone to estrogen, coupled with all the environmental estrogen, that causes adverse effects, such as prostate cancer, not the testosterone in and of itself.

For many years the media has presented testosterone as a steroid that is illegal to take. The testosterone-is-bad debacle was played out in courtrooms and on the nightly news—there was even a cover story in Sports Illustrated.[6]

The results of overuse of testosterone—doping with it—was very much in the news. Many baby boomers remember the Barry Bonds and Roger Clemens takedown attempt in living color. Upon examining the men who were doping, their skin was shown to be bright red, the result of highly dilated veins from lifting heavy weights. Dopers usually have peanut testicles and a small penis—many of them are sterile. They have temper tantrums and eat enormous amounts of food, mostly protein. There is hair loss, and often severe acne, especially on their backs. Their workout schedule is Olympian in nature, and their emotions seem intense and dominant—these men have really short fuses.

There are many reasons for cardiomegaly (big heart), but when the chest x-ray of a man in the emergency room reveals an enlarged heart in a fellow who needs oxygen to breathe, is really red, enormous, and sort of manic, this man will most likely die of congestive heart failure or a heart attack as the result of doping.

To be clear, replacing declining levels of testosterone with the lowest possible dose of bio-identical hormones *under medical supervision* is not doping.

THOMAS'S INTEREST IN TESTOSTERONE

Thomas had read about recent findings out of Harvard Medical School indicating that it's not the testosterone to be feared, but rather how it breaks down into estrogen-like by-products that pose a risk for various cancers, prostate in particular. He understood that it is imperative to have regular blood testing to make sure the testosterone dose is sufficient to be beneficial without converting to estrogen. Hearing that I prescribe testosterone, Thomas came to me for treatment due to his reduced libido, diminished erections, lack of energy, and feeling that he was developing fat around his midsection.

After a thorough exam, I started him on a 100 mg testosterone injection every five days, then every four days. The dose was lowered to 80 mg due to an acne breakout. I also started him on 50 mg of DHEA. I continued the T at 80 mg every three to four days. Soon after, blood tests indicated that the dose was too high, so it was adjusted down to 60 mg, 40 mg, and finally 20 mg, which was determined to be the proper dose. At this level, the acne breakout stopped.

During an interview, Thomas stated that he thought his therapy had the potential to cure every age-related male issue: libido, erection issues, fat around the middle, executive powers, and stamina. To his disappointment, however, his erectile-dysfunction issue turned out to be more psychological, as it did not resolve with the use of testosterone. Testosterone is a libido booster and performance enhancer as long as there are no psychological issues. If there is performance anxiety, guilt issues, intimacy issues, new-woman issues, or any of the other psychological reasons for erectile dysfunction or premature ejaculation, testosterone will not likely do much, unless, perhaps, there is some placebo effect.

Reducing the amount of belly fat was probably the most noticeable benefit. This may not work for everyone, especially if you have an extra large belly. Being thin to begin with, the decrease in flab was very noticeable on Thomas's body; it was confirmed by a high-tech scale that measures fat content.

He stated that he always feels rather confident, so it was hard to tell if the testosterone had an effect on his executive skills. He noticed no increased level of aggression.

So how did it go overall? Thomas noticed that he had high-quality morning and nighttime erections for the first time in years. He wasn't sure if it was the therapy or the fact that he was involved romantically with a new woman. Because there are so many components to sex, it may be difficult for some to tell what testosterone therapy is actually accomplishing, but the end result was gratifying to him and he was happy that he had decided to do the therapy.

It is important to understand that testosterone is *not* a cure-all and that there are exceptions to the norm. There are guys with lots of testosterone who are very fat (usually, testosterone prevents redistribution of fat to the belly). There are guys with lots of testosterone who have sexual difficulties (guys with high testosterone levels are generally considered sexual animals). There are guys in prison with low testosterone (too much testosterone is usually associated with aggression).

It takes a commitment to living a healthful life, along with testosterone therapy to achieve the results you are looking for. Testosterone is not a magic bullet. While it will elevate libido, you may need a boost to function found with Viagra.

Men usually expect their general practitioners to provide testosterone prescriptions. If your doctor is not well-versed in the subject of testosterone supplementation (and many are not), the first thing he/

she will say when you bring up the subject will be a simple statement that it is dangerous. More specifically, she/he will likely tell you it can cause prostate cancer. In other words, they will probably support this old school of thought.

Once the general practitioner (GP) scares men away from getting testosterone therapy, they usually forget about it. Those more attuned may continue on to their urologist to discuss hormonal needs, but many of these doctors are trained as surgeons, and most are not familiar with testosterone supplementation. Endocrinologists (hormone specialists) usually avoid this area of practice and concentrate on treating diabetes and thyroid disorders instead.

Because of the recent pharmaceutical promotions regarding low testosterone levels, more GPs and urologists than ever are prescribing the testosterone pushed by the pharmacy salespeople.

The big problem with all of these new *experts* in treating low testosterone is that they may not be ordering regular blood tests to make sure their treatment is both safe and effective. They may not know what to do to keep the testosterone from converting to estrogen and other negative consequences; they may not even know how important it is. The best thing would be to find a doctor who is well-versed in managing the entire hormonal cascade. Find an integrative medicine specialist who actually trains in presenting the entire hormonal cascade.

While testosterone supplementation should be available to every man in decline, it isn't. After all, who wouldn't want to slow the aging process, live a more vital life, enhance relationships, and extend sexual prowess into old-age? If offered this package, who would turn it down?

The main reason testosterone supplementation isn't more actively employed is due to the limited number of practitioners who have the knowledge, the time, or the desire to engage in such practice. As noted, there is also fear associated with testosterone and its perceived link to cancer. And finally, due to the cost you don't see everyone flocking to this form of therapy. Unless the man's testosterone blood levels are below normal, it is not covered by most medical insurance, even though the low end of normal is reason to supplement, so it is up to the individual to decide if taking testosterone will be a priority for them.

Testosterone Supplements

Testosterone ads are not just coming from pharmaceutical companies. Supplement companies promote herbs to boost the production of your own testosterone, rather than seeing a doctor for prescription testosterone.

These advertisements are very effective at getting the attention of men *and their wives.* "Testosterone deprivation triggers national wave of male sex woes!" "30 million get ED drugs (like Viagra) that do nothing for their sex drive." "U.S. doctors mistake low testosterone levels for ED and depression."

These ads bring attention to all the symptoms associated with low testosterone. And the big three, *decreased libido, loss of self-confidence,* and *depression* are the ones that loved ones, colleagues, and bosses begin to notice, which can make any man feel even more self-conscious.

Because hormone balance is so critical, if supplements increase testosterone, doing so without the guidance of a doctor to monitor your levels is risky. Regarding effectiveness, generally speaking, herbs and supplements used to increase your testosterone don't increase it enough to make the difference seen with taking actual testosterone. This doesn't mean they won't work for you. If you decide to go the supplement route, make sure you have blood levels of all related hormones tested regularly to see if the supplement is working and to make sure it is not resulting in testosterone being converted into harmful substances.

Effective Supplements for Low Testosterone

Here are some of the supplements you can consider.

- Ginseng. This Asian remedy is also used to improve testosterone levels.[7]

- Horny goat weed (*Epimedium*). This is a plant that grows in the high altitudes of China, Japan, and Korea. It is used in traditional Eastern medicine to enhance sexual performance, eliminate stress, and increase testosterone.[8]

- Maca (*Lepidium meyenii*). This is a plant from Peru, sometimes referred to as Peruvian Viagra. While it seems to enhance sexual behavior, in one study, it did not increase testosterone.[9]

- Tongkat Ali, aka Malaysian ginseng. This is found in the root of the *Eurycoma longfiolia* tree. It helps fight stress and increases the levels of testosterone in the body by stimulating the Leydig cells in the testes.[10]

- Some common supplements, such as zinc[11] and vitamin D,[12] are also known to increase testosterone.

Other Natural Ways to Increase Testosterone

Other natural ways to increase your testosterone without prescriptions involve such things as avoiding sugar,[13] reducing stress,[14] eating healthy fats,[15] losing weight, and exercising.[16]

The Role Estrogen Plays in Testosterone Levels

Have you noticed that aging men have breasts, abdomens that resemble pregnancy, that the V-shaped body is long gone, waists are bigger than hips (one definition of obesity), and that they look puffy? Of course, eating the standard American diet (SAD) does not help, but these changes are often associated with the high levels of estrogen (a female hormone) found in aging men.

Besides testosterone converting to estrogen, other reasons why so many men have high levels of estrogen are related to its presence in food (cattle and chickens are injected with estrogen to make them fatter, just as it does with you). Estrogen is found in the plastics that hold food and water. Deficiencies of zinc and vitamin C (no need to take megadoses) also help convert testosterone to estrogen. The white diet (white salt, white sugar, white flour) often results in low levels of zinc. Belly fat stores estrogen and other inflammatory hormones that convert testosterone into yet more estrogen available to wreak havoc on both men and women.

Other things that convert testosterone to estrogen include insufficient omega 3 fatty acids, drinking too much alcohol, liver dysfunction due to poor diet, certain medications, and surgeries.

Just as too much estrogen is associated with women's cancers, too much estrogen is a bad thing for men as well. It can result in prostate problems (enlargement and even cancer), low libido, and erectile dysfunction. This is why men must periodically have their estrogen levels measured whether or not they are taking testosterone. If a doctor merely tests for testosterone and doesn't regularly monitor your treatment, you may be at risk for developing prostate cancer—not from too much testosterone, but from too much estrogen.

What Estrogen Does to Men

For men, the prime of life is when testosterone levels are at their peak. But testosterone does not work alone, it combines with an enzyme called aromatase to produce estrogens. Men's sexuality depends on having a small amount of estrogen for their brain chemistry to trigger sexual function. And conversely, women need a very small amount of testosterone for their sexual function.

Heretofore, doctors were trained that increased testosterone means increased prostate cancer. However, a review of medical literature "concluded that testosterone therapy is not associated with increases in the rate of prostate cancer, or any other prostate illness." Additionally, no evidence was found that testosterone treatment causes prostate cancer, or that men with higher testosterone levels have higher rates of prostate cancer. In fact, it is noted that prostate cancer increases exactly when the man's testosterone levels decline.[17]

Other researchers claimed that men with enhanced testosterone levels realized improvement in every parameter measured: Their prostate glands decreased in size, their PSA levels lowered, and such urinary symptoms as frequency and urgency all improved.[18]

Please be aware that this does not apply to those of you who are getting your testosterone in gymnasiums, on the Internet, or through other illicit means. Men must work with a physician who is knowledgeable regarding how testosterone can convert into dangerous *stuff* that can cause cancer. This can happen even if you don't take testosterone, as your very own testosterone converts into this same *stuff,* which is why there is this great big fat concern about cancer.

Since testosterone aromatizes (turns into) estrogen in men, could it possibly be that increased estrogen in males is what causes so many prostate problems? That is what European endocrinologists think. One sign that estrogen levels are high is when men look as though they are expecting. Isn't it fun to watch when Dr. Oz measures men's bellies and asks when the baby is due?

It is imperative for men to avoid exposure to estrogen and estrogen-like drugs that have a direct effect on the prostate gland. Women, too, must avoid exposure to excess estrogen that affects breast tissue, the uterus, and the ovaries. One of the most likely environmental effects wreaking havoc with men and women is all of the hormones in the current food supply that work their way into the body. As noted, cows and chickens are routinely injected with hormones to make them plump and tender. These hormones produce much larger animals, and that translates into profits for the farmers. These hormone-tainted meats make people fatter, too, as they develop enhanced appetites for more of these foods. At all cost, try to buy beef and chicken that is raised organically, indicating that neither hormones nor antibiotics are used in their care.

It is also important to be careful about what you store and heat your food in, as this matters every bit as much as the food and drinks inside them. Many plastics leach estrogen-like substances into food, water, and other drinks. Never heat food in plastic containers or cover the container with plastic that touches the food. Use glass instead. Throw away old, scratched, or damaged plastic containers. While BPA and DEHP (chemicals that keep plastics soft and pliable) have been proven to have harmful endocrine-disrupting actions, new research shows that the same type of estrogen-like substances even come off of BPA-free plastics.[19] The bottom line here: Avoid plastic containers—especially if they are warmed or heated.

Benefits of Bio-Identical Testosterone

The Brain—Heart—General Health Connection

Besides helping to eliminate many of the symptoms associated with low T, testosterone converts fat to muscle (with aging, every year you lose a pound of muscle that converts to fat), sharpens memory, improves sleep quality, increases bone density, and improves heart function.

There are more testosterone receptors in the heart and brain than in any other part of the body. The heart is a muscle, and in Europe, testosterone is used as a first-line heart medication.[20]

It is possible that, with proper nutrition, exercise, and replenishment of low T with low-dose bio-identical testosterone, many men would not require so many prescriptions for such things as cholesterol, depression, diabetes, ED, high blood pressure, and sleep disorders.

Bio-Identical Treatment

As stressed repeatedly, the fear of testosterone treatment is related to many years of believing that testosterone caused prostate cancer, a belief no longer held by the most current researchers. As noted, it is the excess estrogen, some of which derives from testosterone conversion, that adversely affects the prostate. It has taken many years for medical practitioners to get the message.

Think about how hormones work for men. You have low testosterone that leads to low libido. When you do try to have sex, there is a good chance you'll experience erectile dysfunction or premature ejaculation, which, in turn, causes low self-esteem and depression that drives you to drink and take drugs to forget all your problems. The drinking and drugs actually make sex more difficult. Eventually, as the level of testosterone declines more and more, you don't care about sex any longer, your executive decision-making powers diminish, there is a redistribution of weight to your midsection, your muscles atrophy, and your energy levels diminish.

It really can work this way and it's not all that uncommon. Many people, including many doctors, say this is a natural part of aging. It most certainly is if you are willing to accept that when your body stops making hormones, you just let it be.

Ask yourself, or ask your doctor, if your body stopped making insulin or thyroid hormone, would they just let it be? The answer is, "Of course not." They might argue that deficiencies of the insulin and thyroid hormones are disease states, and sometimes they are, so medicine found replacements, and as a result, people live better and longer lives. The question here is, for a better quality of life, why not replace anything that's in decline? Without controlling diabetes or thyroid imbalances, you may die. But since you can go on living without sex, replacement of the sex hormones is not deemed necessary by most medical practitioners.

Because of the many interconnected reasons why men become sexless, an analysis of a man's problems requires an understanding of this complexity. A particular focus must be on decreased hormone production (testosterone) because, with advancing age, this is a very important factor that affects most everyone.

In fact, by definition, any and all factors related to men's sexless behavior result in a man who has little interest in sex. He couldn't perform if he wanted to, and feels terrible about stressors in his life, not the least of which are his feelings of inadequacy. Sometimes, if all the symptoms are related to that solitary problem, a single remedy will make him better. Other cases will involve treatment on multiple fronts to get the desired result.

If bio-identical hormone replacement allows for a libido boost that also enables a man to achieve erections, he may no longer be depressed about his condition. Suddenly, this one treatment solves so many problems. If his libido is boosted by hormone therapy, but he can't physically perform due to plumbing issues affected by years of poor diet, drinking, and smoking, in addition to the hormone therapy, he needs to separately address the erectile dysfunction.

If this same person went through psychotherapy for depression, or sex therapy for erectile dysfunction and lost libido, he could work on these problems for years and never get a good result because his doctors never addressed the root cause—in his case, low testosterone and defective plumbing. If he took antidepressants, he could feel less depressed, but never get back in the bedroom since many of those medications severely impair libido and function.

More often than not, psychotherapy is not the complete answer for the sexless marriage. In general, there are way too many people taking the wrong course of treatment, and they never get better. Make sure your doctor figures out all of the problems and treats you appropriately. You really do want to get better.

Men want sex because it is a major biological need grounded in their chemistry, psyche, and genes. It is an important way for them to open their lines of communication. I (RM) tell my women patients this little tidbit: The French have a saying that "many problems are solved on the pillow." And while women may think this is an odd way to communicate, men don't.

Testosterone is *the* primary hormone for men and is responsible for muscle mass development and sexual desire. In much smaller quantities, women also require testosterone to experience a healthy libido.

Testosterone Replacement and Male Andropause

It is rare to find men over forty-five who don't have low testosterone levels. However, if the correct tests are not ordered, a man may never know his true status. Low testosterone generally gets lower with advancing age, and, in time, men experience a kind of male menopause that is affectionately named andropause. The authors like to call it *manpause* as it puts men on pause.

What to Expect with Bio-Identical Testosterone Replacement

With testosterone treatment you usually experience enhanced libido, conversion of fat to muscle, improved oxygenation, blood sugar control, optimal immune function, focused concentration, improved mood, partial protection against SDAT (senile dementia Alzheimer's-type), decreased CVD (cardiovascular disease), lowered blood glucose, decreased insulin requirements, decreased triglycerides, and increased insulin-receptor activity.

The Europeans replace many hormones in the lowest possible *physiologic* doses, not big *pharmacologic* doses. There is a big difference. Pharmacologic doses are large doses required to treat disease states, while physiologic doses are small ones and are based on the body's needs for natural function. Hormone replacement or supplementation is best accomplished with bio-identical compounded hormones, not synthetic hormones or those taken from animals.

Hormones are replaced in a variety of ways. There are testosterone patches as well as creams and gels rubbed on the skin (transdermal), pellets placed under the skin, and injections. Testosterone pills are not recommended because they can cause serious problems with the liver.

Follow-up is important, as the goal is to keep your hormones in physiologically normal ranges and keep you disease-free. That is, at a forty-year-old level, forever, feeling good and being able to perform the way you did back then. The goal is to make you a healthy hot aging man with an edge.

REPLACEMENT DOES THE TRICK

Sam T. is a sixty-two-year-old male in good health and of slender, though muscular, build. Blood tests showed a testosterone level in the low-normal range. His family doctor dismissed the low reading by saying it was in the *normal range.* When Sam questioned his doctor about testosterone treatment, he was told there are too many risks associated with hormone replacement, especially the risk of prostate cancer, and the subject was dropped.

Sam decided to go ahead with testosterone treatments anyway, and when he did, the main adverse reaction he noticed was acne. Not a simple breakout, but rather deep pimples called cystic acne, which stopped when he was given a reduced dose. It's no wonder young men have all those pimples at puberty. The good news is that they go away in time as the testosterone levels off.

Sam's main purpose of getting the testosterone was to be able to get erections on demand. His expectations were not met, however, because it turned out that the past was clicking at his heels. In further discussions with his doctor, it came out that his inability to have an erection on demand was due to his being upset by his wife's withholding sex and having affairs. But Sam's plight had a happy ending because, in time, he was able to overcome his problem with the help of testosterone, some *emotional* surgery, and the loving ministrations of a new woman.

Cancer Fears with Testosterone Treatments

Regarding testosterone therapy, the breakthrough change in the thinking was first reported in 2010 by Dr. Abraham Morgentaler, a Harvard Medical School urologist. His research and views are best explained in his book, *Testosterone for Life.*[21] Essentially, he states how the myth that testosterone causes prostate cancer is based on flawed research concerning one single case of the disease. To the contrary, low testosterone is actually associated with a high prostate-cancer rate and, as such, is detrimental to men's health.

If your doctor is not aware of this recent research, you may want to consider finding someone who is versed in the latest body of medical science and not stuck in outdated ideas.

Doping with Testosterone

What happened was that the word steroid got relegated to the category of being something bad. Although there are many steroids, testosterone included, that are necessary for the vital functions of life, anything to excess has the potential to be bad, and doping with testosterone is bad.

Men who dope with testosterone take herculean amounts of injected testosterone daily. Men dope with testosterone to be dominant, both physically and mentally. Most men who dope utilize a program called stacking, which is the intramuscular injection of various forms of legal and illegal testosterone. These doses are strong and excessive, in short, abusive.

Men who dope usually stand out in a crowd. They are enormous. They don't know that they look grotesque because they have bigorexia, which is the opposite of the eating disorder anorexia, usually associated with women.

Then there is the death thing. Meteorically high testosterone creates hypertrophy (enlargement) of all muscles. The heart is a muscle. The left ventricle of the heart becomes so enlarged and hard (LVH— left ventricular hypertrophy) that it is not able to pump blood from the heart to the rest of the body.

The Bottom Line

There are a few things you can do to increase your testosterone and decrease your exposure to environmental estrogen.

Watch what you eat. No one expects you to never eat beef or chicken again; however, unless you find a place that sells or serves organic chicken and and beef, it will be difficult to avoid estrogen exposure from your foods. You can stick to vegetables and wild fish at restaurants, and buy the organic stuff for your home cooking. Basically, follow the dietary recommendations in chapter 7, All About Men, in the section on Diet for a Healthy Prostate.

For food and drink, try to avoid plastic bottles and containers, and use glass.

Take testosterone under the care of a knowledgeable physician. As much as you may want to be *all natural,* bear in mind that it is *all natural* to grow weak and old. The only effective way to stay young, from a hormonal point of view, is to supplement when the chemical is no longer produced in your body at sufficient levels to replace what is gone. This is the most definitive way to keep you from becoming your aged father.

Exercise, not fanatically, but consider walking almost daily. Moving, and not sitting too much are crucial. Is sitting the new smoking? Are we ruining our health by maintaining a sedentary life in front of our computers and television sets?

Reduce stress by trying to reduce the easy things that cause your stress. Don't be afraid to take a break on a regular basis throughout the day to clear your mind and stretch.

9

Physical Issues

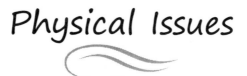

Your General Health

YOUR HEALTH AND PHYSICAL CONDITION HAVE MAJOR IMPACT ON your sexuality, as does the health and physical condition of your spouse. If you *let yourself go,* you are the problem that can lead to a sexless marriage, just as if he/she let himself/herself go, he/she is the problem.[1]

General Heath and Sexual Health

Coronary Heart Disease

Men with coronary artery disease (CAD)—clogged arteries that feed the heart—have clogged blood vessels everywhere, not just the heart. Since erection is dependent on blood flowing into and out of the penis, those clogged blood vessels will make erections weaker, or result in erectile dysfunction.[2] In some cases, erectile dysfunction may be the first sign of CAD and a visit to your doctor should not be ignored if you experience erectile dysfunction, even if you have no interest in sex.

Besides slowing blood flow to the penis, CAD usually results in decreased blood flow everywhere, which is a big cause of decreased stamina, a condition that hinders those who want to engage in sex. Fear of imminent heart attack is another matter to manage since CAD can lead to a myocardial infarction—heart attack. If you have a fragile heart, there is the real fear that overexertion in the bedroom could kill.

Some people with heart problems may lose confidence and worry. This can cause a type of ED that is referred to as psychological erectile dysfunction. It is usually grounded in fear, anxiety, and/or guilt.

Estrogen provides a heart-protective effect in women. That is why they have less heart disease than men of similar age. However, once they reach menopause, women can develop similar cardiac risks due to a decrease in their estrogen production. They have to be concerned with heart attacks and strokes once they reach, and advance through, menopause, unless they take hormone therapy to restore youthful levels of protective estrogen.

The heart and lung health issues affecting stamina affect women and men equally. With less energy and endurance, engaging in sexual activity may be difficult. Sexual activity can lead to a shortness of breath. Using a prescription inhaler before sex and finding less active positions for sexual activity can help.[3] To insure vital lung capacity and health avoid environmental toxins and stop smoking, NOW. Smoking is probably the number-one self-induced destroyer of health.

Diabetes Mellitus

Diabetes is another disease that affects every blood vessel in the body. Over time, if your diabetes is not under control, the risk of heart disease, stroke, blindness, loss of toes and feet, and erectile dysfunction becomes more likely. A yearly checkup will often uncover diabetes before it has done so much damage. Keeping slim and avoiding excessive carbohydrates, especially the refined ones, in your diet help prevent diabetes.

Cancer

Cancer affects sexuality on many levels. There are changes in physical appearance, the result of surgery or radiation, as well as psychosocial responses, including grief, depression, and anxiety. Besides anxiety and depression, survivors of ovarian cancer may experience sexual dysfunction and identity disturbance.[4]

Cancer that requires penile, prostate, rectal, or testicular surgery may negatively affect sexual activity. Such medications as leuprolide can interfere with libido, as can a fear of physical harm from sexual activity. It may be best to resume sexual activity slowly. Consider beginning with a massage and mutual masturbation to help overcome any performance anxiety.[5]

Obesity

Obesity is probably the *nutshell health issue*. In a nutshell, if you are obese, you are at major risk for all the deadly physical factors affecting sex, as well as the threat of an increasing risk for cancer, debilitating back and joint injuries, diabetes, heart attacks, and strokes. If you do only one thing to help your life in general, and your sex life specifically, that will be to avoid obesity. If you are already there, you must fix it, or you will very likely place burdens on your relationship with your mate and die younger than if you maintain an appropriate weight.

Keeping Healthy

Prevention includes proper diet and cessation of all activities that promote cancer, heart disease, and the rest of the lifestyle diseases, such as smoking, poor diet/overeating, sedentary life style, poor sleep, and avoiding routine medical exams (there's a reason they are called lifestyle diseases).

Diet

Diet includes a moderate intake of fat, dairy, and red meat, increased wild-caught fish, consumption of complex carbohydrates (whole grains, not white flour and white rice) in smaller quantities, and increased fruits (whole fruits, not processed juices) and vegetables. To avoid the toxins, hormones, and antibiotics that now contaminate food, especially meats, chicken, and fish. Try to purchase organic meats and chicken. Because diet is so important in preventing major illnesses, aging, and decline, this recommendation should become an integral part of your new way of living.

Exercise

Regular exercise builds the system that delivers healing oxygen to every cell in your body. It lubricates your joints, preventing and improving arthritis. It feeds your brain, slowing the progress of dementia by up to fifty percent; it strengthens your immune system, and it builds bone and muscle mass, contributing to good health in myriad ways.

Sleep

Sleep. Seven to eight hours per night of restful sleep contributes to weight loss, mental clarity, and overall immune function.

Stress

Stress reduction. Cortisol has been referenced numerous times in this book as a negative, unhealthy stress hormone when it is produced in large amounts for a long time. Meditation, deep breathing, yoga, Tai Chi, laughter, relaxation, and good sex all contribute to the decline of cortisol levels.

Sexual Peak—Both Physical and Psychological

It is often stated that men and women reach sexual peaks at different ages. There is much confusion about sexual peak. To help understand the issue, realize that there are two types of sexual peak: biological and psychological. The two forces, mind and body, interact and dictate sexual desire, performance, and frequency.

Biological Peak

The biological peak relates to the highest levels of hormones being produced, which occurs around puberty. You would expect the highest levels of sexual desire and activity to coincide with this peak, but the availability of mates and knowing how to perform may not be all that great at that young age, given the little amount of experience that accompanies the biological peak.

Psychological Peak

Psychological peak is related to the way sexual desire and activity may be altered as a result of the individual's psyche. Factors affecting the psychological aspects of sex include mental state, experience, societal dictates, and stress levels associated with jobs, relationships, and raising children.

If society says sex is bad for young girls, which it has for many generations, then the chances for sexual activity and desire may be stunted during that age. If society tells young girls that sex is fine at any age (think more today than in the past), then sexual activities may rise for that age group. Understand that when a peak is described as an age, that age is just an average. Don't expect to wake up hitting your peak on that particular birthday.

As a result of what can be described as a new sexual revolution, psychological sexual peaks have changed radically. To determine if your psychological sexual peak is in line with others your age, you have to make an assessment based on the generational divide that sees older women reaching their psychological peaks (age thirty-six) many years after their biological peaks (age sixteen) as they escape societal dictates regarding female sexuality from their youth and become more experienced. In essence, those women who were inhibited in sexuality at their biological peak often break free of the societal taboo and engage in a form of sexual freedom that they missed early on.

The Timing of Sexual Peaks

As young girls today become sexually active near age sixteen (their biological peak), unencumbered by societal taboos, they may actually show a *decline* in sexuality by age thirty-six, just like the guys have for generations. Their need to explore sexuality at thirty-six may not be necessary, as they already finished much of their exploration in their teens and twenties just like the guys did.

One common description is that men hit their sexual peak between sixteen and eighteen, while women reach theirs at thirty.[6] The authors believe this describes the biological peak for guys and the psychological peak for gals, thus apples are not being compared to apples. As noted, the biological peak defines the time that hormone levels are at their highest, usually around eighteen for males and a year or so younger for females, maybe sixteen.

Since the psychological peak for male sexuality is not really discussed or described, it is an educated conjecture on the part of the authors that guys reach theirs at around twenty-four. The basis for this assertion is that their hormones are still churning, they've had a chance for a good amount of experience, but the rigors of career, the ordeal of raising children, and the ravages of a sexless marriage have not yet affected them. In essence, the fellow at twenty-four years of age knows what he's doing and is enjoying it more than at his biological peak where inexperience may be keeping him from maximum performance and enjoyment.

If hormones can be maintained at youthful levels, there is no reason that sex can't be enjoyed more and more in later years where performances continue well into ages never before considered highly sexual.

Due to the altered mores of American society, it is predicted that the sexual peaks for both men and women will come in line with each other, and this will mean that both groups will experience the peaks and valleys of sexuality more in unison than in years past.

How does the sexual peak relate to the sexless marriage? It is imperative to consider where you and your partner are related to sexual peak. If a man or woman who is in decline suddenly finds that their mate is more sexual, this can result in incompatibilities.

You are wise to understand that one or the other of the couple may need more or less attention and sexual activity based on sexual peak. By understanding that societal and religious dictates also play a role in the reception or repudiation of sexual activity, you will be better able to identify what areas need work.

10

Psychological Issues

Your Mental Condition

A HEALTHY RELATIONSHIP IS THE SUM OF ITS PARTS. IT IS NOT just sex. Good satisfying sex is the result of a deeper connection—one built on mutual respect, good communication, compassion for each other, and abiding affection. These are the building blocks of love. Some things can get in the way, such as mental or physical illness, differing ethics or morals, or a lack of anything on the list of building blocks. Take away that base, and the relationship could be on shaky ground. This chapter will briefly look at the ways that mental infirmities can make for the sexless marriage and worse.

Psychology of Sexuality for Men

Men are usually heart-wrenchingly desirous of sexually pleasing their partner, but ironically, one of the few human endeavors that fails to improve with concentration and determination is creating an erection. For some men, the solution is to use Viagra as a psych med, since they know their performance issues are often in their minds.

Erectile Dysfunction as a Psychological Problem

Masters and Johnson did important work on sexual dysfunction in the sixties. Unfortunately, their findings that most men with erectile dysfunction (ED) have a psychological problem set progress back a bit.² Medicine is dynamic, not static. With much research it has been learned that most men with ED have a physical basis for their problem (clogged blood vessels, prostate issues), but some do have a psychological cause for ED. The mind is the largest sexual organ in the body, and marital conflict, depression, fear, guilt, stress, and anxiety can manifest as ED. Anxiety releases adrenaline, which makes the penile blood vessels constrict like a twisted hose. Worrying if your penis will respond intensifies the situation. Even Viagra and the other ED medications don't always work.

If ED is psychological in origin, please know that there is an option in the form of penile injections, which always work. The needle is very, very tiny and there is a self-injector.

Depression

This is the other major issue in men that could affect their libido as well as their performance.₁ Depression is often something men don't want to admit, address or even realize they have, but when depressed, some men really don't have any desire to do much of anything. Without question, deep and/or longstanding depression needs the help of a professional.

Psychology of Sexuality for Women

Psychosexually speaking, women may experience three major issues.

- Depression
- Loss of libido
- Frigidity/anxiety/fear of sex

Frigidity and anxiety over sexual activities are usually associated with serious issues. A surprising number of women have been molested, and have experienced incest or rape in their lifetimes. Few have gotten the help they need to overcome it. The event may have been hidden from their conscious memories, particularly when it happened in early childhood, and events in the present may trigger the body memory and cause them to fear sexual union. These issues require professional help, though often, no one likes to talk about getting that help.

Hypoactive sexual desire disorder (HSDD). HSDD is defined as a lack or absence of sexual fantasies and lack of desire for sexual activity. To be regarded as a disorder, it must cause patient distress or problems with relationships. Interestingly, there are subtypes where HSDD can be a generalized lack of desire, or situational, meaning that desire exists but not for the current partner. The appropriate understanding of the type of HSDD is required to resolve the problems.[3]

Managing Female Sexual Anxiety

Women don't have to come to the party with a loaded sex organ, but even so, for some women, their psychological and physical issues are just as compelling as those of the men.

When confronted with psychosexual difficulties, a conversation is in order. In this case, the guys have to get the ball rolling because a frigid or depressed woman will not usually start this conversation. If she is willing to try to work on the problem with you, you have an obligation to go slowly with deep care and understanding.

Perhaps some cuddling or light petting can be incorporated into each evening, with the strictest understanding that it will not lead to sex for a reasonable period of time. Based on a predetermined schedule, heavier petting, and then sexual exploration can begin. The sexual activities progress until sexual union is hopefully enjoyed by both parties. If there is opposition to any such program, or if progress is stalled, it's time to speak with a professional psychologist or sex therapist.

Mental Conditions—Mental Infirmities

Mental infirmities can make for the sexless marriage, and worse. A person's mental condition is a major factor in how they see the world as well as how they interact with others. The range of mental health issues that impact relationships extends from mild depression that may see couples less engaged in conversation or activities to full-blown major depression, personality disorders, schizophrenia, or bipolar disorder, with extreme manic and depressive episodes. If you suspect that you or your partner may have some form of mental illness and neither of you have been diagnosed, seek help. Needless to say, your sour mood or inability to enjoy life will negatively impact your relationship. Anger and jealousy destroy the foundation of trust and quickly erode relationships. There are effective medication-based or non-medication strategies available; there's no reason to endure, or cause your partner to endure, the pain and distress of mental challenges that could possibly destroy your relationship when help is available.

Mental illness of any type, from mild to severe, is an *illness,* not a failure on your part or that of your spouse. Seek help. Learning to control your temper, seeking help for depression and other mental disorders goes a long way toward maintaining a good relationship and avoiding the sexless marriage.

Many people are in denial and discount, or make light of, their disorders. Mood swings, antisocial behaviors, belligerence, and physical attacks can bring a relationship to the brink of dissolution. Further, many people with mental problems tend to self-medicate with alcohol, prescription drugs, or illicit drugs that only complicate the matters.

It is extremely difficult to admit that you are the one with the problem. Often a person will blame others and never look in the mirror to see how they contribute. If your spouse keeps blaming you and you keep blaming him/her, and neither of you are capable of taking responsibility, it's time for couples therapy and perhaps individual therapy.

Don't expect your life to improve without help if one or the other has a mental disorder. You will only relive the same negativity over and over. The arguing, the withholding of sex, and the loss of any viable passion will lead to the sexless marriage. If you are already there, you have to do something about it. Granted it is difficult to make this happen because you have to confront your mate and have the very serious discussion that if they will not join you in therapy to improve the relationship, you may have to leave.

The same reasons why people stay together are the reasons why this conversation and taking action is so difficult. If your mate is the violent type, having this conversation is dangerous. You should seek the advice and counsel of a professional who handles these cases, usually found at a local shelter. Money is always an issue where neither side wishes to have a radical change in lifestyle, which is inevitable when couples get divorced.

Money concerns may also work in your favor to find solutions, once the reluctant spouse realizes he/she will lose half their wealth because they were unwilling to try and fix the relationship. Money is a great motivator.

Making sure that your mental condition is not the result of diminished hormone levels cannot be overlooked. Decreased levels of the sex hormones can result in mental issues that are often mistaken for primary mental problems. Getting a blood test to make sure your hormone levels are in order may help you to find an appropriate treatment that may not be psychotherapy.

Mood, Depression, and Mental Illness

Depression is the most common mental illness, and the incidence increases with age. In the United States depression affects more than 58 million children and adults annually.4

Depression that can affect the marriage, or any relationship, comes in many flavors and exists in many degrees.

Mild depression can lead to lack of interest or participation in activities. This reduces the opportunities to bond with a mate, and others, resulting in isolation and loneliness that serves to make the depression worse.

In severe cases, depression can result in complete withdrawal and eventual institutionalization. Initially, it seems innocuous enough, since it often begins with mood changes, social isolation, and less sex. All of this may be associated with business pressures, PMS, and andropause or menopause, depending on the age of onset.

Depression can be the result of many causes, even low testosterone or low estrogen. Make sure you get a through medical exam before starting psychotherapy. No need to bark up the wrong tree. If depression goes untreated, it may end in sexless relationships and worse.

Depression may manifest itself as weight gain or loss.[5] The change in body shape and form can become a stressor in a relationship. While in an ideal world, acceptance of negative changes would be wonderful for the one changing for the worse, in reality, when depression leads to eating disorders, the changes can become so exaggerated that sexual attraction is lost.

Frustration and low tolerance to stress are not listed in the annals of psychology as mental conditions, but they can cause the same relationship consequences as depression, which is often the underlying cause. Several general responses to frustration and low tolerance for life's trials are: disrespectful utterances continuously directed towards the partner; passive aggressive behavior; or yelling and screaming. If not held in check, these can be devastating to the partner who may feel abused. In time, the couple may eventually develop deeper rifts that progress into full-blown contempt and animosity.

Learning to control your temper, manage stress, and seek help for depression and other mental disorders goes a long way toward maintaining a good relationship and avoiding the sexless marriage.

Personality Disorders

There are many types of personality disorders that can affect your life. Two in particular are the *sociopath* and the *narcissist*. While they are different, both are characterized by the person being more interested in their own happiness, comfort, needs, and desires than anyone else's in the world.

Sociopaths

Sociopaths have no regard for the feelings and welfare of others. They are more inclined to be controllers and unfaithful to the extreme. People with this disorder may exhibit high-risk sexual and criminal behavior.

Once you realize you have married or cohabited with a sociopath, there isn't much you can do to change them. You should get the help of a professional who can guide you through your dilemma. One option is to get the sociopath to enter therapy, though this is not very likely to help as they often refuse treatment, or may go along for the ride to appease you, with no intention of changing—recovery rates are low. Alternatively, you can live with them while trying to control the risks, or leave them and move on with your life.

Narcissists

The term narcissist is probably used way too much in our culture, or perhaps we are all a bunch of narcissists. The designation is not to be used for the typical self-centered individual, though that's one of narcissism's principle traits. In actuality, the term used by psychologists, Narcissistic Personality Disorder, refers to an extreme case of preoccupation with self, personal adequacy, power, prestige, and vanity. This personality type is generally unaware of the destructive nature of their problem, either concerning themselves or in their dealings with others. Sound like somebody you know? Before you rush to classify everyone with this disorder, however, you should know it is estimated that only *one percent* of the population is affected by this excessive form of egocentrism.

Dealing with an egotist is bad enough and you should have figured this out before you became partners. If you are stuck in a relationship with a narcissist, getting them into treatment is in order. But a problem arises here because these people generally do not think they *have* a problem and, as such, are not inclined to get treatment. If the narcissism becomes too destructive, you may have to leave the relationship.

Personal and Behavioral Issues

THERE ARE MANY BEHAVIORS AS WELL AS PERSONAL ISSUES THAT do not belong in relationships, especially intimate relationships, if you expect them to thrive for many years. The distinction between personal and behavior concerns is not always clear. For simplicity, assume that personal issues are things you don't readily control (like lost love or financial problems), while behavioral issues are things you have under your control (like neglecting your mate or withholding sex when it is done to punish).

Here we explore some of the most destructive personal and behavioral problems and learn how to remedy them.

Maintaining Good Health for Good Sexual Activity

Without good health, it becomes difficult, and at times impossible, to engage in healthful sexual activity. The very reason for leading a lifestyle grounded in prevention as a means of staying healthy, is to keep you from getting to the point of no return, which would mean no sex. That should be a good motivation, but sadly many people give little thought to prevention while they are still healthy and able to function.

Naturally, you have a major responsibility to yourself, your mate, and your family to stay healthy for reasons beyond sex. It is wise do everything you can to avoid succumbing to the major preventable diseases (hypertension, heart disease, and diabetes) that ruin your ability to provide for your family. No one can promise you won't get sick and die, but if you don't take care of yourself by making the appropriate lifestyle changes, your neglect is a time bomb for a stroke, a heart attack, diabetes, and cancer, dooming you to see your health destroy many aspects of your life.

Hormone replacement is never going to be a replacement for a healthy diet, regular exercise, quality sleep, quitting smoking, and well-controlled stress. The strategies in this book are designed to work *with* a healthy lifestyle, not instead of it.

Basically, any disease that ruins your lungs, heart, and blood vessels will affect your sex life. When lungs don't function optimally, your body doesn't get oxygen or expel toxic waste in the form of gases, so it backs up in your blood and clogs the vessels. When blood vessels are clogged, you have less blood, oxygen, and nutrients getting to the vital organs, the penis being one of those organs vital to sex.

A big downside of certain types of heart disease is that it prevents men from taking oral erectile dysfunction medications (Viagra). The priority here is to keep your heart healthy.

Breast cancer patients may experience postmenopausal symptoms from chemotherapy and the use of tamoxifen. Use of lubricants may be required for sexual activity to enhance the experience.[1]

The Busyness Factor—Your Busy Life

A good relationship for most people means spending time together. While it doesn't have to be a 24/7 bonding, there is the need for balance that requires spending quality time with your mate. Quite often, the *busyness factor* ruins many relationships.

Think back to the times you were the happiest with your mate, and try to recapture the activities that were once important and promoted that happiness. Because people get busier as life moves forward, it is too easy to stop going to the movies, stop taking a Sunday ride to *anywhere,* stop so many of the activities that once defined your relationship. Once the fun, bonding activities are gone, only to be replaced by the stress-producing effects of hard work, career goals, and raising a family, it's easy to see how a sexless marriage can sneak up on you.

Just as scheduling and appointments play a major role in business affairs, your marital affairs require the same. If sex is no longer spontaneous, and if enjoyable time together has faded from your *to-do list,* you may need to set aside time in a schedule that includes such activities.

There is a catch-twenty-two element to the busyness factor as it relates to relationships. Many people highly value success and money and the lifestyle it can afford. After all, couples to whom these things matter most usually live in the biggest houses and drive the best cars. They dine at the finest restaurants and sport some of the most beautiful jewelry, while their children go to the finest schools. However, achieving success and money usually takes a great deal of hard work and requires time outside the home and away from home and family. Relationships often suffer. There are many mates who, while enjoying the fruits, incessantly complain about how they never spend time together, never go on vacations, and have seen a decline in their sexual relations. Even if money and success do not follow the hard work—too many people work multiple jobs just to make ends meet— the time and subsequent exhaustion demands a lot of a relationship.

It's not always possible to change the stressors that cause time away from home and partner, but each person must be aware of how they respond to them. Constant complaining is destructive to a relationship. It chips away at any joy, pride of accomplishment, teamwork, or self-esteem that existed before. Both partners become unhappy and that unhappiness grows as the partner who feels attacked avoids the complainer. This avoidance can either be physically, by seeking reasons not to be there, or mentally, by shutting down and tuning out. Problem drinking can occur, as well as drug use—escape by any means. The relationship is destroyed.

It doesn't have to be this way. Whether the partner is driven by success and the desire for more wealth, or by the basic financial pressures of eking out a living in this difficult world, the other partner would be wise to seek out positive, two-way communications instead of destructive complaining and nit-picking. There is a cliché that says, "Walk a mile in his shoes." That means put yourself in his or her place and try to see the world as he or she is seeing it, with the pressures and demands being faced and how you are helping or harming the situation. This is compassion.

Time together needs to be valued in a relationship, no matter how much or how little. Look for ways to appreciate that time and the person you love. If there has been a lot of animosity, try and remember back to a time when you were happy and in love.

What did you do then? What can you do now? First, turn off the TV and cell phone. Go for a walk. Hold hands. Enjoy a meal. How about a romantic sexy evening together? It is certainly a stressbuster. The intimacy involved could reignite the closeness you once felt.

If you don't want to continue the negativity, or end up in a sexless marriage, or worse, each spouse must value and focus on quality time spent together.

Sadly, in youth, relationships are often based on chemistry and lust and have little understanding of compatibility based on deeper issues, such as work ethic, responsibility, career goals, and dependency on others to feel fulfilled. In time, differences and incompatibilities fester and result in relationships that drift apart. If you are feeling any strains in your relationship, it is imperative to make an assessment of the various issues before the sexless marriage results.

Realistically speaking, you are not going to get an A-type personality to think less about business concerns, nor are you going to make a dependent person happy spending time alone. There are, however, compromises and solutions that should be considered. These involve working with your strengths and minimizing weaknesses, as well as finding substitutes that may help you to feel fulfilled.

Since the original bond in love relationships is often grounded in sexuality, it is important to keep it going. What often happens is that, as sex is relegated to an unimportant activity, you find that the one common bond that glued you together is no longer present.

Taking Steps to Relieve the Busyness Factor

The first step is to try and make your busy mate happy in ways that require the least amount of time. Act sexy, hug your mate, and hold his/her hand when going places. Act like you are happy to see her/him when he/she comes home

Do the special little things you used to in the courting stages. Initiate sex and be slightly persistent even when they are too tired. If some petting is employed, it may move toward fulfillment This has to become part of your life if you want to keep the relationship fresh.

If nothing above seems to help, it's time to have a talk. You have to confront your mate in a non-threatening manner. Let him/her know how you feel, and offer solutions rather than just recognizing and complaining about the problem. Point out that you have been trying to get the relationship back on track, by saying, for example, "I've been trying to be more understanding and affectionate, but you seem to be pushing me away."

In the discussion with your mate, you must be forthright and able to make sure there are no underlying reasons for the downturn in the relationship, i.e. make sure it is the busyness factor and not lost libido, an illicit affair, or mental health issues, such as depression, that are the root causes (and are addressed in other chapters).

If one of you is so busy that you can't make time to fix the relationship, it will fail. If one of you is so dependent on being with the other all the time and is unwilling to find a life in such healthy endeavors as hobbies, charity work, friends, family, perhaps even a job for fulfillment, then this will also cause the relationship to fail. It takes real effort on the part of both parties to make a relationship work, but the payoff is a relationship that regains the magic that started it in the first place.

Do understand that many people get lost in their work because the relationship turned sour. You must do a serious self-assessment to see why you are hiding in your work, or why your mate is hiding in his/her work. If you have let yourself go with weight gain, poor hygiene, or self-destructive habits and are no longer physically attractive to your mate, if you are often depressed and never in the mood to engage in sex, or if you don't treat your mate with kindness and respect, you have an altogether different issue. It's not the busyness factor—it's *you*. If you don't make the changes necessary to fix the problem, your relationship is over, whether your mate leaves you or just stays for convenience.

Taking Action by Fixing Yourself Up

This is something you must do. Even if you, individually or collectively, let the relationship decline too far and it's over, fixing up yourself has its rewards. You will look better, feel better, and be a much better mate for your new love interest if you choose that route in the future. If you don't fix yourself up, your future is likely going to be full of illness and loneliness. Which case sounds better to you?

Familiarity and Boredom

Boredom in a relationship may be another way of saying *you have fallen out of love* with your partner. Somehow, over the years you have grown apart. Your mate no longer excites you, either sexually or socially, and seems to get on your nerves for just about any reason. This boredom, or falling out of love, is a major reason so many relationships fail.

For some couples, being together a great deal of the time works well. It allows them to know each other and grow together with common interests. On the flip side, however, there is, of course, the old adage—*familiarity breeds contempt*. Too much time together may push people apart. And while another adage states that *absence makes the heart grow fonder,* pay heed as well to the one that says *absence may make the heart wander*. Finding a balance is necessary to keep your relationship healthy.

Based on surveys of German students from ages nineteen to thirty-five, Dietrich Klunsmann stated that sexual activity and satisfaction declined in women and men as the duration of the relationship increased; sexual desire only declines in women; desire for tenderness declines in men and rises in women.[2] Furthermore, he told *The New York Times Magazine* that women who don't live with their partners retained their desire more than women who do.[3] Esther Perel, a couples therapist states that, "Eroticism requires distance."[4] Lori Brotto, a psychologist who works extensively with hypoactive sexual desire disorder (HSDD) patients, ponders the thought that the condition may be boredom rather than libido.[5]

Fending Off Boredom and Resentment

Besides making sure that your hormone levels are working to keep you interested sexually, another way to keep boredom from happening has to do with keeping some space between yourselves for healthy growth, but not so much that you grow apart. You should neither smother nor neglect your partner.

In the early stages of relationships, especially for those with wildly active hormones boosting desire, being apart is unfathomable. The same couple whose hormones have long passed optimal levels and who have had many years to get on each other's nerves may get to the point that being together becomes a burden. If sex is their only connection and it is no longer important, the quality of their relationship is doomed.

Much resentment builds against the mate who puts career, friends, activities, or hobbies in the forefront and neglects their partner. This resentment can go beyond the marital relationship, as the children are often neglected as well.

Figure out where you fit in the spectrum of time spent with your partner. You have to be able to see any extremes, and that takes real vision. Talk to your mate about his/her feelings regarding time spent together. You may be surprised to find that while you think all is well, they may want to be with you more or less than the current situation. Attempt to reach some compromise and make efforts to get the balance needed to keep familiarity from breeding contempt and to keep the heart from wandering.

Familiarity may turn into boredom. A multitude of therapists ponder the ever-perplexing problem associated with waning sexual desire. They debate the cause from a psychological understanding. While there is most certainly a psychological component to boredom in the bedroom, overlooking the diminished hormonal element may be the hidden cause in many problem relationships. It appears that not too many therapists start with a blood test to determine the possible hormonal cause of such boredom. Hypersexual, young married couples rarely get bored with their sexual partners while their hormones are churning.

It is important to look for a mate who is both interesting and interested—interested in growing as an individual and as a couple. Stagnation in a relationship only works when both parties remain stagnant and don't care.

In youth, it is difficult to predict where you may be twenty or thirty years into your relationship. Quite often people marry for hormonal/sexual reasons or to have a family. While these may be great reasons to propagate the species, with aging they don't work as well toward compatibility and something more in common is needed.

A big reason to search for a new mate is that people don't grow together as they age. They grow apart. For women, as an example, the sports-loving, beer-drinking, carefree nature you fell for as a twenty-something may become repulsive as your interests in culture and educational pursuits flourish at forty-something.

These differences are often difficult to manage and may become irreconcilable as time marches on. But since all good things take a lot of effort, strive to find common interests. If you find yourself growing apart, you both must make efforts to spend more, not less, time together. Try to take courses together. If your partner is interested in dance, religion, language, cars, home décor, fashion, theater, or other such interests, make an effort to become involved. You need your space at times, but too much space leads to the dissolution of the marriage after enough time of being sexless and separate has passed.

Two Relationship Killing Behaviors

Withholding Sex Syndrome (WSS)

The purpose of defining withholding sex and neglecting your partner as *syndromes* is to emphasize that these behaviors can most certainly result in serious *physical* and *psychological* symptoms. All too often the medical community doesn't recognize that appropriate interpersonal relationships, as they may relate to health, are important and not just personal issues. Negative behaviors can definitely affect a partner's health.

When it is used too often, withholding sex, a common destructive behavior, can result in what can best be described as withholding-sex syndrome (WSS)—A syndrome is a group of symptoms characteristic of a specific disorder or disease. WSS usually causes both psychological and physical symptoms and results in a high degree of failed relationships.

This negative behavior can be perpetrated by either sex, though it is a device much more used by women, especially by those who don't like sex or can take it or leave it.

Women, especially, take note of this: All those times you sent your mate to sleep rejecting attempts to connect may have been no big deal to you, but you can be sure your mate was not happy. Just the fact that he continues to try indicates that sex is important to him. His resentment may have built up over the years, resulting in that explosive announcement, "I'm leaving you," which blindsides you because you were oblivious to the root cause.

Sex is often important, very important, and it is something every smart prostitute knows well. If you don't take care of your man, she will. And if you're lucky, it's just the prostitute taking care of your man and not some other woman.

If people really enjoy sex, it is not likely to be withheld. When withholding sex is done by a woman, it is for one of several reasons. She could be turned off to sex or find sex painful for physical reasons. She may withhold sex to punish her husband for some real or perceived transgression, or merely because she is in a bad mood, often associated with hormonal changes or depression/mental illness. She could also be involved in an affair.

Those men affected by their mates withholding sex may regress and avoid sex. Or they may find other outlets that include pornography, masturbation, prostitution, and illicit affairs, which can result in feelings of guilt and depression.

Combine less testosterone, seen as the man ages, with sexual rejection and you have a perfect formula for erectile dysfunction and lost libido.

Withholding sex is not just a woman's thing. Men can be vindictive and manipulative in their motives for withholding sex, though they are less inclined to do so. Men withholding sex is more likely related to depression, stress, erectile dysfunction, or illicit affairs.

In cases where the woman is much more sexual, the man who has a lower libido may be inclined to withhold sex when he becomes angry because the woman does something that upsets him. The diminished libido may just stunt his desire to engage for no apparent reason. Those women affected by their mates withholding sex may find other outlets that include masturbation and illicit affairs, which may result in guilt and depression. Women rarely resort to pornography or prostitution.

Depending on the cause of the WSS, getting better may be difficult. Withholding sex could be rooted in passive aggressive behavior that may be part of the personality of your mate; not easily fixed.[6] You may need to get counseling or psychological help. You could open the dialog at a time when anger is not in the air and explain to your mate that withholding sex is unacceptable in your relationship and that something must be done. Suggesting the need for professional help is your offer to find a remedy. Now it's in your mate's court, and you let him/her come back to you with an offer. If your mate refuses to acknowledge that a problem exists, then you have a big problem.

People who can't understand or see their failings can't fix them. Now you have to decide if you move on or stay frustrated. Trying to mend the fence without professional help often sees a brief reprieve, only to have the behavior repeated. If you didn't address withholding sex early in your relationship, you will very likely need professional help.

There is nothing good to come from withholding sex. If you or your spouse is using this as a tool to control behavior, it must stop. Get help otherwise expect frustration, divorce, or both.

When a mate withholds sex it often leads to frustration, anger, and ultimately contempt for the partner. According to Dr. John Gottman, a leading marriage researcher who spent years studying marriages, contempt is the best predictor of failed relationships.[7] If there is any one thing in relationships that breeds contempt, withholding sex is paramount on that list. Being let down from sexual excitement too many times finds some men unable to get aroused for fear that the carpet will be pulled out yet again.

When a woman withholds sex too often, her partner can develop both physical and psychological symptoms. The associated anger, frustration, and stress can lead to anxiety, depression, heart disease, high blood pressure, poor sleep, prostate problems, psychological erectile dysfunction, weight gain, and strokes. [8,9,10]

Men can play this game, too. Many similar symptoms associated with sexually deprived men can be seen in women. These include anxiety, depression, high blood pressure, heart disease, poor sleep, sexual dysfunction (vaginal atrophy), strokes, and weight gain.

Neglected Partner Syndrome (NPS)

The other profoundly negative behavior most likely to cause anger, frustration, stress, and ultimately divorce is neglecting the partner. And just as withholding sex results in a group of associated physical and/or psychological symptoms, making it a syndrome, so does neglecting a partner.

Described here for the first time, neglected partner syndrome (NPS) is all about a relationship where one mate no longer approaches his or her partner to engage in most activities, including sexual activity. NPS is common with a waning sex drive because the sexual attraction that keeps people together bonded is diminished or gone.

It's not just women, either. Men have to be careful too, just like women. While your neglected woman is not likely to hunt for a gigolo, she may very well hunt for the attention of a man willing to service her both emotionally and sexually, a deed that could end up with him living in your house while you still have to pay many of the bills in the form of alimony. It's no longer just a man's world. Both women and men need to be attentive to the emotional, social and sexual needs of their partners because sex plays an important role in relationships.

Over a period of years, changing interests may find that one of you has little in common with your partner. A partner who espouses negativity, is depressed, or who has let themselves go physically, spiritually, and socially is not the type of person with whom you want to spend time. The busyness factor, as already discussed, finds one partner being neglected as well.

NPS is not normally seen early on in a relationship when hormones are raging—newness adds a level of intrigue, and you haven't had time to become bored or fall out of love. NPS is associated with the same physical and psychological symptoms seen in the withholding sex syndrome, including anxiety, depression, heart disease, high blood pressure, poor sleep, prostate and vaginal problems, sexual dysfunction, strokes, and weight gain, all highly correlated with the anger, frustration, and stress associated with the decline of intimacy.

NPS is not to be confused with a man or woman engaged in an affair. Even though the affair results in the same symptoms, in NPS there is a lack of time or desire to engage with the partner, not a distraction associated with another love interest.

At best, NPS results in a shallow relationship devoid of much affection, and it may lead to the sexless marriage, depression (if it isn't already part of the cause), illicit love affairs, and divorce.

Other Causes of NPS

- Physical changes. These can make a mate less desirable and may be associated with NPS, especially if the neglecting mate has become hypersensitive to reasonable changes that occur naturally with aging. If you don't take care of yourself, you may become the neglected mate who is undesirable.

- Attitude. This can also play a role in NPS. You can't be miserable and testy to your partner too often and not expect him/her to withdraw from you.

- Hormones. These play a big role in that your partner may no longer lust after you as she/he did in earlier years. Once the sex drive is diminished, it doesn't take much to decide upon spending time with your partner versus watching the ballgame, going out with friends, or drowning yourself in work. If your partner has not experienced the same decline in sexual desire, he/she will beg for sex only so long before losing interest or finding it elsewhere.

- Taking things for granted. Besides all the reasons offered to explain NPS, there is one other that is difficult to affix because it is part of human nature—*we take things for granted.* Ask Floridians if they are in awe of, or even notice, the palm trees and they will look at you like you are nuts. It is human nature to become complacent about things that are ever-present. Steak every night gets to be a bore.

Just about anything done all the time, or to excess, may become unappreciated and eventually neglected.

Remedies for NPS—Ways To Prevent the Sexless Marriage

- Effort. To avoid complacency, showing appreciation for everything you have in a relationship is worth all the effort it takes. Good things come to those who work their behinds off to achieve them. Improving the quality of your relationship takes focus and effort. It must be important to you. Your partner must be important to you. If you are not willing to work for it, all the hormones and/or therapy in the world will not change your sexless marriage.

- Sex quality and variety. While the *quality* of sex is always a challenge as people and the relationship age, if the quality can be kept up, the *quantity* will surely flourish. People tend to repeat things they like, that make them happy, and that feel good.

For many, sex is *plain vanilla,* and that's just fine if both partners like vanilla. No need to read further if your sexual practice is good for both parties—if you are sexually compatible. For others though, there may be concerns about sexual practices that could have a serious effect on the relationship. These concerns may be coming from the partner who is afraid to ask for what she/he needs to turn on, or they may be coming from the other partner in the form of a refusal. It is hoped that by the time your marriage has become sexless, you have some inkling of what your partner liked when things were good. It is also possible that, without communicating such desires, there are other things your mate might want that you are not aware of.

GROWTH OF SELF AND YOUR MATE

Make-Up Sex

From the *Urban Dictionary* 1. Rough and extremely gratifying sex had after an argument. 2. After a couple has an argument and decides to settle it with sexual relations. The best sex there is.

Who invented make-up sex? Whoever it was, they probably also invented things like fire and the wheel, but wanted to make an even more important contribution to humanity so they came up with *make-up sex.*

If world leaders could figure out how to have make-up sex, chances are there would be no more wars.

Make-up sex is the physical act that is used to fix the effects of an argument. It is an important tool that helps bond those who have just engaged in an uncomfortable and sometimes hostile quarrel.[11]

But, in the sexless marriage, this tool is *gone.* Without make-up sex, conflicts large and small may be more difficult to put to rest. This is one tool you must try to keep in the bedroom. Of course when desire is gone, there can be no make-up sex. It must be brought back.

The way make-up sex works has a lot to do with the bonding experience, and it is very much grounded in hormonal responses. After an argument, libidinal needs seem supercharged, so instead of being physically aggressive, sexual release offers an acceptable and welcome alternative. In both men and women, the release of the bonding hormone, oxytocin—sometimes called the love hormone—calms and connects the combatants upon release after intimacy.

Assuming you still have some desire and your marriage is not completely sexless, you never want to refuse make-up sex.

There are, however, some rules to make-up sex that must be followed.

When engaging in make-up sex, neither party can assume that he/she won the argument. It's not like, "Now that you see it my way, I want sex." That doesn't work. Instead, the one initiating sex has two options.

They can apologize if they realized they were wrong once they had time to calm down and think about the situation.

Or they can offer a general apology for making their mate feel bad, "I'm so sorry we got into that argument. The last thing I want to do is make you feel bad. I realize we have a difference of opinion, and I want to respect your opinion and review all this later when we are both feeling better."

The mate receiving this form of apology must follow the rules as well. He or she must be grateful that their mate is feeling bad and wants to fix things. Since they are trying to make up with the most powerful stress-relieving tool in the world—sex—this is not the time to continue the argument.

Now go for some gentle kisses and wait for a response. As the receiver, you become gracious and say, "I know you never want to hurt me and I'm sorry you feel bad. I agree, let's talk about this later."

It's that simple. Make-up sex is not about winning the argument. It's about connecting on a higher level that tells your partner, "I love you, even when we argue." Now you escalate the kissing and you're ready to roll—that is under the covers.

Sex Make-Up—Grooming

Neglected grooming may be both the *cause* and *effect* of the sexless marriage. Obviously, poor grooming may cause couples to avoid sexual encounters. It may also be the effect if you are no longer having sex because the relationship has been corroding from negligence, anger, illness, the busyness factor, or hormonal deficiencies. In that type of marriage, there isn't much reason to dress up for encounters with your mate.

Without sex makeup (our new term and effort at wordplay to accompany the term make up sex), and more broadly defined here as *grooming/hygiene,* the couple slides one step closer to the sexless marriage. Other than debilitating depression, there's no reason you shouldn't make every effort to be clean and look good, and maybe even go out of your way to pretend you are trying to attract your mate by your appearance. The competition is out there and you can be sure they're trying to look their best.

As men age, they may decide to grow a beard, usually to hide the newly noticed double chin. This may work well to soothe the ego of the aging warrior, but it may be a real turnoff to his partner. Discuss significant changes before you act, like before you grow a beard, and don't be afraid to ask if she likes beards. You have to make your concerns known, and you have to decide who has the *bigger need* in these types of situations. If you truly can't kiss your guy with a beard, he should be told, because the more you force yourself in disgust, the more you may pull away altogether. Of course, if he grew the beard for his *new* mate, he'll be happy that you stay away.

The areas of grooming that concern both of you have to do with hair growth and care, body cleanliness, and oral hygiene. Make every effort to keep your hair clean and neat. It should smell fresh and not be oily or filled with dandruff flakes. You should shower as often as necessary to avoid ever having body odor. Bathroom wipes provide a much fresher state of affairs than toilet paper that merely moves smelly feces around the area that is closest to the *playground*. There is nothing more of a turnoff than engaging in oral sex with someone who is not *squeaky clean*.

Ideally, it's good to shower right before engaging in sexual activity. If your mate likes to be spontaneous and surprise you, this isn't always possible, but if you can shower, it makes for a much nicer encounter. Interestingly, people engaging in illicit affairs usually make sure they are *immaculately clean*, hygienically speaking.

In general, each side should ask what the other likes and try to make it happen. And don't be afraid to compliment often. Compliments help your mate know what pleases you. After all, you may have a tendency to criticize, so try using sugar as well.

Listening

Listening is not very hard to do. Just shut up and listen. Let them express themselves *without interruption*. Then tell them you heard what they had to say by actually repeating several of the points they made. Now it's your turn to tell them your concerns and address theirs. They, too, have to listen politely, without interruption. They repeat some of the points you made to show they heard you, and then it's their turn again. As silly as this method seems, all too often people don't listen. The other person feels as if they have *no voice*, a great psychological term that is often tossed around in therapy. You must each have a voice in the relationship. You must each feel you are heard. You must each make efforts to not only hear your mate but to act upon the stated needs.[12]

Negativity

If couples make a pact to have no negativity between them, they have the potential to fall in love again. That means no shrill comments, no judgment, and no harmful behaviors. Employing the no-negativity edict in your marriage may also mean you will realize you don't have anything to say to each other unless it is filled with bile, with the immediate result that you may not speak for quite a while. But then a miracle may happen, and one of you will develop a sense of curiosity toward the other, start asking questions, and truly be interested in the answer even if it doesn't fit your worldview. The glaciers between you will slowly melt, and sexual communion will begin.

Identifying the Problem

The following will help you identify what has gone wrong with your relationship and start a dialog with your mate.

Honesty is necessary for any relationship to survive the inevitability of change and the forces of complacency. Some partners remain the same for decades. Others change constantly.

Many of the problems are so complex, there may be several areas that need attention. There are also those issues that are so intertwined that, by fixing one problem, you may resolve all the others.

Hormones are responsible for mental health, controlling weight, helping you sleep, overall general health, and a host of other aspects of your life. Sexual activity is best between healthy, well-rested couples, who can perform physically and mentally. While it's not always that simple, you must identify all factors ruining your marriage and fix them before it's too late. A patch here and there will not get long-term results, while getting to the root cause improves your chances for the complete recovery of a broken relationship. Fix the root problem and the others may come along for the ride.

When asked about sexual frequency, many folks have to give it deep thought. The math isn't really that difficult, it's the realization of how often they have sex compared to how often they thought they had sex that is the shocker. "Gee, I thought we did it more than that."

No matter how you do the numbers, there is clearly a decline of sexual activity as people age. If you weren't happy with the frequency of your sex life in your fifties, you're probably not going to like what the future holds. But for those who don't like sex, they will probably enjoy their age-related sexual decline.

Everyone ages at different rates depending upon genes and the various behaviors that affect aging. The government even has statistics that tell, on average, how long people are going to live.[13] You can read studies about medicine, sociology, anthropology, human behavior, and aging, and you will find there's a pattern that people pretty much follow. Puberty arrives at a similar range of ages; sexual behaviors begin at average ages; and even certain illnesses and conditions show up at predictable times in life. Generally speaking, people participate in physical activities for average periods of time, then change that pattern due to a decline. Most people just can't keep up with the demands of certain activities. There aren't too many sixty-year-old men playing tackle football, and few sixty-year-old women still have dance recitals.

If you marry or engage in regular sexual activity in your late teen years and continue until the age of fifty-nine you can expect, on average, forty years of reasonable quality and frequency of sexual activity. The question arises: how to increase this span of activity by ten, twenty, and even thirty years?

Since the universal and biggest factor in waning sexual desire and activity is hormonal, then bio-identical hormone replacement is the most effective way to extend this life-enhancing activity. The main point of this book is to define the various problems associated with relationships and how the natural decline in the chemicals that make up humans are often the root cause of these problems.

You have many choices as you go through life. You can let the natural order of things play out, or you can take charge and do something to remain vital in all aspects of your being by proper diet, supplementation, and exercise, and the appropriate replacement of the chemicals that wear out.

Go up to just about any person in their late eighties or older and pat them on the back (gently). You will feel the telltale sign of aging and hormonal decline. Their shoulder blades and other bones are often all you feel. They usually walk slowly and with questionable balance. Their skin is thin, their bones are brittle, and their minds don't have the acuity of just a decade before.

But you do have choices. You can become this old person, or you can maintain a level of vitality that was not available in years past. Bio-identical hormone replacement doesn't guarantee extended life, but it does offer an enhanced quality of life—and that includes your sex life. You do have choices.

Assessing Relationship Problems

Before you can resolve relationship issues, you need to assess them with a cold eye. This is important for everyone to do as they age, to make sure they are growing as a result of their union. Finding a cure for a broken marriage or relationship becomes more difficult when too much time passes with no commitment to finding a cure. Many people avoid finding a remedy altogether, and the result often ends poorly. The divorce rate speaks volumes.

If your mate doesn't think there's a problem, you have a real challenge.

Now you need the facts. You need to gently point out that the frequency of your encounters is not in line with the *average*. And while the goal is not to be average, that's when you quote from the figures we provided, and your discussion is underway. You may also suggest that your mate read this book to understand where you are coming from. Perhaps, highlighting a few relevant parts would be a quick way to understand your concerns.

Number comparisons are stark and work best with men. Women don't always respond to numbers as well as they do with feelings. If it's the guy who has to confront his partner, the goal is to use *I feel* language to be heard, and once heard, then listen—the greatest gift anyone can receive.

Depending on how bad your situation has gotten, you may be in for some surprises like, "My sexual frequency is just fine as long as you don't come home early, because that's when I see Hans, my tennis coach."

There are a number of men and women whose spouses come out

of the closet, and they are shocked. Maybe there were clues they ignored. Given their sexual preference for a person of the same sex, many were very content to be in the sexless marriage, while their partners blamed being sexless on getting older. They may have been fine with it, but obviously, their partners, who were still in the dark as to their sexual orientation, were not.

Resolving Relationship Issues

All the many possibilities to assess and resolve relationship issues are reviewed in this book. Open your eyes to see that relationships are two-way streets—each of you needs sexual fulfillment and attention to differing extents. If you are not attuned to the needs and differences of your partner you can't resolve relationship issues.

Hormones and Sex

Hormones are what make people want to have sex (they stimulate the libido), not porno films, or great perfume, or anything else. If you have significantly diminished hormones, you aren't going to desire sex, regardless of any outside stimulation. Alternatively, you can have great hormones, but if the plumbing isn't working, you aren't having any sex.

If you're depressed, you may not often be in the mood for sex. The degree of depression dictates the impact on mood. With mild depression, you may do your marital duty by going along for the ride, but won't likely initiate the act—or enjoy it. Does any of this sound familiar?

Some people say sex isn't everything. Generally speaking, however, the people who say this are not having any satisfying sex and they may not be experiencing the joy that marriage can provide when sexual activities are included.

Exploring Remedies for Diminished Desire

It is important to explore some of the remedies for the sexless marriage and see why there is no need to live life without sex if you don't wish to. When you explore the connection between the many factors that make you sexual, that will help you see how to keep them functioning properly.

Without hormones churning desire, there is little more that can be done to fix a non-sexual union short of taking a good acting class, pretending to want to have sex and pretending to enjoy it once engaged in the act. While women can do their wifely duty without desire, performance by men devoid of desire is not going to happen without Popsicle sticks and duct tape. Women can fake it, men can't.

Even with hormonal balance, before you can expect desire to be part of the equation, consideration must be give to the mental state, social interaction, physical connection unrelated to sex, physical condition, time allowance for the relationship to thrive and alone time for recovery from overload one or both partners may feel.

What may have been desirable in youth can change—values and tastes often evolve. Sometimes one partner changes and becomes more emotionally stable, spiritually conscious, and cognitively expansive. If the other partner remains the same twenty-five-year-old person, the bonding that sex provides becomes less important. Add the decline in most every hormone and sex may become a distant memory you cherish.

Replenishing Hormones and More

The subject of hormone replacement pops up all through the book because it is the essence of fixing so many relationships. Replenishing hormones is a valuable remedy that will help fix many sexless marriages, but there is so much more. Perhaps it's time to work on self-growth, regain your former leanness, and continue to be attractive for your mate. Being considerate to your mate, listening, and spending time together will also kindle fire. A friend once stated, "It's more important to be heard than anything." Being heard requires mono-tasking and often results in a renewed desire to bond sexually.

The Decline of Taboos

The decline of taboos is a force going on in many parts of the world, and in America in particular. Taboos have been eroding from one culture to the next, with American culture leading the way and being emulated by so many others. Cultural trends are very rather powerful and affect everyone, sometimes in unexpected ways. The taboos of adultery, pornography, and prostitution that once helped stabilize the institution of marriage—and kept divorce rates low—have seen their day.

The benefit of making divorce so available makes sense. Too many people have been living miserable lives and now they can escape without feeling the wrath of societal condemnation. The downside of eliminating the divorce taboo, besides the affect on the nuclear family, may be seen in the cavalier reasons for divorce and the rejection of trying to work at the relationship.

These four former taboos can seriously affect your marriage. If you keep your head in the sand, you may find yourself in a withered relationship that only continues because of these now-accessible outlets.

It appears there are those who are oblivious and can't fathom that there are outlets for the mates of those who withhold sex or neglect to show their partners affection and appreciation. If prostitution and pornography are multi-billion dollar industries, you have to ask yourself, who is engaging in these outlets? Is it your partner? Is your head in the sand? Have the lack of taboos that once protected institutions and condemned certain behaviors affected your marriage?

For a healthy marriage, you would be wise to make sure your mate has no reason to engage in behaviors that are no longer taboo. A mate who is sexually satisfied, fulfilled, and even satiated is not looking for interests outside the home.

Grooming to Attract Desire

Although the subject of grooming has already popped up several times (including in the earlier section on sex makeup in this chapter) it is an issue that cannot be overlooked when it comes to desire. Unless your mate has a fetish, poor grooming is a turnoff. The stench of sweat and body odor, bad breath, greasy hair, or an unkempt, crusty beard or pubic region, are distasteful to most people. Take a shower, brush and floss your teeth. If you have rotten teeth or gums, see a dentist; if you have vaginal discharge or odor, go to the doctor because that is not normal. Open sores, bumps, scabs, malodorous discharges, and passing gas (try some simethicone, it works for most people) are just as unattractive to your partner as they sound now, as you are reading this list. And no one wants to kiss you if your breath smells like that of a camel.

When couples date, they are likely to engage in their pristine grooming. They shower, style their hair, use deodorant and cologne, and women often adorn their faces with makeup. Many people go all out, wearing their best outfits, pressed and ready. It's all part of the mating game. Not too many would expect success in dating if they didn't make some efforts to put their best foot forward.

Sometimes one partner is doing just fine in the grooming department and their mate is being neglectful. This is certainly a problem and needs to be discussed before it becomes an issue. The partner most upset by the lack of grooming has to step up and begin the dialog. While difficult, the opening begins with, "We have to talk . . ."

If you're too embarrassed to talk about grooming directly, then make a special effort to notice and comment whenever your mate does do something positive in terms of dress and hygiene. See if they are not attracted by the reward of a sincere compliment to repeat or expand the behavior. They may have been feeling invisible, unwanted, or unloved, and the act of noticing them in a positive way may stimulate their desire to care about their appearance.

Another option is to make concerted and noticeable efforts to look nice for your mate. When they notice and make a comment, it becomes easy to say, "I want to feel like we're dating again. I want to dress up and go on a date once in awhile and I want you to join me."

If this doesn't add a spark to your mate's behavior, it may be because they are depressed, and that's a whole different, and more difficult, story.

As people age, some find grooming burdensome, or they become oblivious to their looks. Some think it doesn't matter any longer since they're already married. Others become tired, sick, or depressed to such an extent that commonly acceptable grooming is neglected. Then there are those who get so busy with life they no longer take the time required to stay well groomed.

Women are usually more attuned to grooming than men. Poorly groomed men may be depressed, but they are usually too busy or don't care, while women who go around poorly groomed are more likely depressed or ill. Here are some pointers in the grooming department.

Teeth should be brushed after meals, but if you don't do that, at least make sure you brush well right before you begin kissing. Try chewing gum as it increases salivary flow for cleansing and it freshens your breath. If you have foul breath that doesn't respond to brushing, flossing, and mouthwash, see your dentist to see if there are gum problems, cavities, or food catching between your teeth. Certain medical conditions may be the cause of bad breath, and this requires treatment by your family doctor.

Use cologne or perfumes if your mate enjoys them, but don't go crazy—a little goes a long way. A nicely scented body moisturizer might be all you need.

The Libido

Hormones may churn desire, but libido (the sex drive) is what makes sex happen. At least one of the partners has to want to be sexual, and they need a mate willing to at least participate if their libido is not in sync with that of their partner's. If both partners are without libido, forget about it, it's not going to happen.

They may be closely related but there is a distinction between desire and libido. Libido feeds the desire for one thing—*sex*. Libido is raw, lustful, instinctual, and primal, whereas desire can be much more cerebral. You can desire to go to the movies or buy something nice, but libido is what makes you lust for sexual union/intimate communion.

For whoever has the stronger libido, it is important that their mates learn to emancipate their sexuality so as to enjoy blissful union as a couple in a successful and happy relationship. Many couples with differing libidos lead frustrated lives that may end in extramarital affairs as well as dissolution of the relationship emotionally and/or physically in divorce.

If your mate wants to engage in sex, you should not refuse too many times because all you are doing is setting your partner up for a libido-deprived state. You do this too much, and you may discover he or she has found a new outlet for getting into a libido-satisfied state.

There is much information here about why you may not be feeling responsive to your mate and what to do about it so you don't have to win the Academy Award for acting. Much of this book delves into the psychological and hormonal reasons for neglecting partners If you want a good union, work toward keeping both parties in balance.

Does libido fade in time? Can you look forward to a time when neither of you will want to engage in sex because the desire is gone? In years past, a diminished libido was a foregone conclusion. As hormones faded, so did the physical ability to have sex as well as the desire (libido).

Now, however, thanks to longer, healthier life spans, hormone replacement, medications for erectile and vaginal dysfunction, and emerging information, couples can remain sexual long into old age. This is especially true if both parties care for themselves and each other and are willing to learn and grow.

Here's a nice story relating to this: An eighty-five-year-old patient told me (RM) she still loves to lay in bed with her husband and feel his skin. She still loves the way he smells, the way he understands her quirks, the way he continues to learn new things and be interesting, and the way he smiles at her.

The Not-Listening Problem

When deciding to try and fix marital problems by engaging the services of a family therapist, listening may come up as one of the bigger complaints many couples have. Problems associated with marital difficulties often have roots in the fact that people don't listen to their mate's concerns, needs, and desires.

If you want to avoid a sexless marriage, you have to listen to one another. All too often mates' talk falls on deaf ears, or mates don't even get the chance to talk or express themselves. One of the most common and important lessons that therapists try to teach their couples is how to listen to one another. If you do end up in therapy, there's a good chance you'll pay a lot of money to learn these skills.

If you want to fix the sexless marriage, you have to start listening. Sometimes what you need to listen to doesn't even make a sound. A sexless marriage doesn't make a sound, yet it rings loud in the psyche of either partner who wants to engage in sex, but is frustrated by the lack thereof. If you don't listen to that message, the relationship is usually doomed.

The fact that the relationship is sexless requires dialog. You cannot be embarrassed or afraid to confront the message. If you repeatedly broach the subject and it is made light of by your partner, you have to demand (in a nice way) that you both seek out a therapist trained in helping with your particular issues. This allows the dialog to begin, and it offers a referee who can keep the dialog grounded and healthy.

If you don't have the luxury of retaining the services of a therapist, you can try the simple methods noted above. But you both have to be on board with wanting to resolve problems. If there is major resistance, your problems go far deeper than having developed the complacency that resulted in your being unable to hear each other. If either or both of you have no interest in listening to one another, you may need to recognize that your relationship is over, and it's time to move on.

The Not-Talking Problem

With time and loss of intimate communion, the not-talking situation opens the possibility to search for a conversation with someone else. Giving energy to a new relationship withdraws energy from the original relationship. Perhaps the new relationship is only an emotional relationship, but it does have the potential to damage or end the marriage.

At times, you need to engage in meaningful conversation, and even not-so-meaningful blather to keep your mate feeling a part of the team.

Compatibility

Relationships are all about compatibility. And when it comes to sex, it's best to make sure the two of you are compatible. If you start out compatible, you have to recognize that may change over time, with many factors coming into play. If your relationship is worth salvaging, you may have to work extra hard to maintain compatibility levels, or you may have to seek treatment if the issues are beyond your ability to solve.

If the relationship neglects the importance of sexual compatibility, this often finds the couple separating once the differences become too burdensome.

Contentment

For most people, there are averages regarding the amount of sex in their relationship and that average changes with time. As long as both of you are content with your sex life, there is no problem. What many people don't understand is that when their mate is not happy, they may not tell them, or may have told them in many subtle ways for years and they weren't listening.

Neglect

It's not just women, either. Men have to be careful too, just like women. While your neglected woman is not likely to hunt for a gigolo, she may very well hunt for the attention of a man willing to service her both emotionally *and* sexually, a deed that could end up with him living in your house while you still have to pay many of the bills in the form of alimony. It's no longer just a man's world. Both women and men need to be attentive to the sexual needs of their partners because sex plays an important role in relationships.

Determining a Mate's Potential Sexuality

It's not really that easy, nor is it effective, to come out with a written test to determine your potential mate's sexuality. In the course of conversations about sex, however, you may pick up on those little hints that tell you what's not so easy to ask. In the beginning of a relationship, having sex several times a week is common. If your mate makes a statement like, "I hope you don't expect to go on like this once we're married," it says a lot. And this is okay if you, too, feel it may be too often and realize it's not expected to continue at this pace. If, however, you need this level of sexual intimacy on an ongoing basis, this may not be the person for you. Keep your ears open for little hints as to your mate's desires and needs.

It is also important to understand that the stated frequency of sexual encounters can and does change as people age. Just because a twenty-year-old husband or bride wants to have sex five times a week, doesn't mean that, by fifty, desire is going to stay the same.

Alternative Sexual Practices

If a marriage has become sexless, and it not physical or hormonal, there may be other reasons that require your attention. Could it be a sexual disconnect? Could what one partner requires for fulfillment be confusing or even repulsive to the other?

Make a date where you meet your mate somewhere for an encounter and make love in a hotel room like you have just met. The preparation—showering, grooming, dressing up in sexy underwear, and meeting at a club or bar—adds an element of excitement, unless, when you arrive, you find your spouse walking off with another person.

Have sex in rooms other than your bedroom. This can be more spontaneous and exciting than the same old routine. Providing your mate with a sensual massage, complete with exotic lotions and vibrators may provide the kind of pleasure you've been missing and that never grows old. Take a course together on massage technique to get good at providing each other with this form of erotic pleasure.

Sexual perversion is relative, and as such, you must recognize that if you bring anything of this nature to the bedroom, it may be repulsive and a major turnoff to your partner, only making things worse for a relationship already in trouble. So be careful, but don't be afraid to explore other activities that may enhance your relationship.

Some alternative sexual practices are as simple as dressing up and role playing. Some involve a power exchange, as in bondage and discipline (B&D) or the more intense sadism and masochism (S&M). A little spanking or being tied up on the bed with some old neckties (as long as the partner feels absolutely safe) is a far cry from beating someone with a whip or urinating on them, so some education is in order. There are many sources to learn about the variety of practices that were once called sexual deviations. You can check for sex books and videos on Amazon. Quality sex-education books and videos address many options.

When introducing new ideas into the bedroom, it is imperative to keep an open mind and start slow. A little time may allow for new ideas to become fun and not threatening. Don't come home and announce how you would like to have a sex harness installed on the ceiling that allows you to hang over the bed like a waiting chandelier. It may be smarter to start with the suggestion of having mirrors installed over the bed so you may watch each other while passionately embracing.

Reading sexy novels together and watching pornography, also together, may offer an enhancement to the libido, as well as offering some chance for a dialog: "Would you like to try that?" Try not to show disappointment if you get the response: "Are you out of your mind?" This at least tells you where the boundaries lie.

You are wise to respect your mate's desires and boundaries. There is nothing more destructive to sexual relationships than to have one partner dread certain activities. If one partner is partial to anal sexual activities and the other is repulsed, this has to either be struck from the list or the repulsed partner needs to consider some compromise. If sex toys or pornography are a turnoff, make the effort to please your partner by avoiding them.

What happens when you find your partner doesn't want to try anything different and is turned off by *all* of your suggestions? It may be time to seek counseling or consult a sex therapist. You may have a compatibility problem and it may be insurmountable, but if the relationship has value to you, it is worth seeking professional help before throwing in the towel.

You want the quality of your sex to stay at a high level, as this will lead to an increased quantity of sex and better bonding. It should allow your relationship to never become sexless and should allow you to grow old together.

Interests and Activities in Common

As time marches on and sexuality diminishes in a relationship, you are wise to find ways to reignite the fire, but you should have other things besides sex to do together. Watching ball games alone every night or going out dancing with your friends every night is not the way to nurture your relationship unless both of you like such activities and engage in them together.

When sex was important, you never refused to go to the theater as long as there was a hopeful expectation of sex at the end of the night. Now you send your husband/wife to a ballgame or the theater with his or her friends while you do what you want to do. Too much of this behavior doesn't bode well for your relationship.

The winners in the relationship game usually have things they like to do together with ever present laugther. Whether it's golf, bridge, antiquing, dancing, shopping, watching sports, or NASCAR, Try to find a mate who does things you like to do or at least makes an effort. You do the same.

Do both of you like to travel, shop, exercise, watch movies, go to the theater, engage in sports, or watch sports? Go through the list of all possible interests and activities and make sure the two of you like to do things together. If there are activities that only one of you enjoys, that doesn't need to be a deal breaker unless the other partner doesn't have their own activities and feels left out—or maybe even becomes jealous of the person with whom he/she shares that activity. Communication is the key to understanding what your prospective mate feels and needs, as well as what you feel and need. The last thing you want is to be a Sunday afternoon football widow or a night out with the ladies widower.

The importance of common interests can't be overemphasized. There is always the probability that one or both of you will change and develop new interests. Your compatibility may change over time, but if you start out with too many differences, your chance of failing is much greater.

The remedies may not be easy, but they are a necessity if you want your sex life back. Only you can identify the problems in your relationship and learn ways to fix them. There is hope.

Medication Issues

Unfortunately, many drugs treat the symptoms and do nothing to heal the cause. Furthermore, the medications you may already be taking for various ailments can affect the libido and sexual performance.

These issues need to be addressed. An example of such a problem is the decreased sexual desire, in both men and women, associated with taking any of the group of antidepressants called SSRIs (selective serotonin reuptake inhibitors), which include Prozac, Zoloft, Paxil, and a host of new generation antidepressants.[14] These medications, which may be necessary for some cases of depression, can send desire out the window and make it incredibly difficult to achieve an erection or reach climax. SSRIs in low doses are often prescribed to help men who experience premature ejaculation, so, if anything, they may slow or prevent orgasm.[15]

Certain medications for high blood pressure may cause erectile dysfunction.[16] These include some of the water pills (hydrochlorothiazide, aka HCTZ) and beta blockers (like Atenolol). Blood pressure medications that are less likely to cause ED include ACE inhibitors, alpha-blockers, and calcium channel blockers—ARBs (angiotensin II receptor blockers) and may actually *improve* sexual function. If you feel your prescription medicine may be hindering desire or performance in your relationship, you may want to discuss these options with your doctor. Do not, however, stop or delay taking medications prescribed for high blood pressure. Hypertension is called the silent killer and can cause a lot of damage to your vital organs if left untreated.

Balancing Conventional and Alternative Medicine

There is usually a nice balance between conventional medicine and alternative medicine that could serve you well in managing most every ailment, as well as allowing you to function at a higher level than you would without taking a proactive approach to aging. Don't be afraid of supplements or carefully vetted prescription medications. Only you can slow the aging process by making a concerted effort to replace the things your body no longer makes. To avoid getting into trouble with health issues, teach your children to avoid all the bad habits early on or make the appropriate lifestyle changes before good health becomes an impossible task.

Menopause

Although menopause was addressed in Chapter 5, it is worth review-ing here in terms of behavior.

Women transition through menopause in an intricate fashion. After all, women are complicated hormonal life forms that actually make babies. Perimenopause, the time prior to menopause, may result in many changes for up to ten years. Then, menopause seems to appear over a weekend. Women say, "I woke up and was ten pounds heavier and could never lose it," and, "I love my husband, but, if he died, I wouldn't date, nor would I have self relations."

So, in a very short amount of time, women may go from the minor changes of perimenopause (irregular cycles, spotting, heavy bleeding, worsening PMS) to experiencing many of the 150 possible symptoms of menopause.

Managing this problem is tough to do in the usual eight-to-fifteen-minute doctor visit, especially when all that most doctors learned in American medical residency programs was to prescribe the latest synthetic hormone pill. This may cause cancer, and the FDA says you should take the lowest effective dose for the shortest amount of time.[17]

Many women don't feel comfortable telling their doctor the truth about having a litany of menopause-related complaints. If they do, they may not feel their doctor is taking them seriously. The list can go something like this: ....."I have hot flashes, night sweats, day sweats, vaginal dryness, loss of urine when I sneeze or laugh (if I'm still laughing at all), absolutely no interest in sex, an inability to reach orgasm, chronic urinary tract infections, pain with sexual relations, changes in my skin, an inability to lose weight, the sudden appear-ance of a muffin top, and abdominal fullness."

They take a break to catch their breath and continue: "I'm losing hair. I crave junk food even though I know it's bad for me. It takes hours to get to sleep, then, when I finally do, I can't stay asleep. And when I wake up, it takes so many hours to return to sleep that it's time to get up. Then, I'm exhausted. I can't concentrate. I have to make lists for my lists because I can't remember anything. I have a short fuse. I used to be able to regroup, but now, everything seems like a monumental task. Life seems overwhelming and I think, what is the point?"

Their doctor just stares, trying to pick one thing to *fix*.

Of course, not all women have this many symptoms at once, but the sexual symptoms, such as reduced libido, are pretty universal. Without treatment, this person doesn't make for the best company. She is especially not the best partner for sexual relations. Dryness and thinning of the vaginal walls can make sex painful, if not impossible. If guys had sore penises after sex, they might be more sympathetic to this most uncomfortable female change-of-life experience.

At this point, the woman usually receives a prescription for an antidepressant, a sleeping pill, a tranquilizer, and a vaginal lubricant, plus a pill for her bones, which are beginning to look a lot like Swiss cheese. She may also get Ospeneal, a newly approved prescription drug for vaginal dryness and pain. The listed side effects of Ospeneal include hot flashes and sweating, so it may not be a good choice for a woman who is already radiating heat like a supernova. But are these prescriptions really helping the patient? Are they the only answer? No.

Other Reasons for a Dimmed Sex Drive

Besides menopause, there are other reasons, starting at much younger ages, that can result in a diminished libido for a woman and a sexless marriage. These conditions have been around a long time, but more recently doctors have come up with technical-sounding names for all sorts of issues affecting women's sexuality in order to better describe and study the problems.

Although men experience depression and other mental illnesses, they nevertheless still find moodiness and irrational behaviors rather disruptive. Double standard? Of course. But when these behaviors are present too often in a spouse or lover, or if the degree becomes too noxious, or sex gets withheld as a result of said behaviors, the man may withdraw or seek an escape. He may get lost in work, hobbies, or television, or engage in excessive drinking, pornography, prostitution, or affairs.

PMS (pre-menstrual syndrome) is the cause of many sexless relationships, and much frustration and angst, both for the women experiencing the symptoms and the men who have to cope with them. Marriages may fail under the strain.

Physical problems associated with the sexless marriage may require treatment by qualified urologists or gynecologists. Intervention can be as simple as counseling in the use of appropriate lubricants, or as complex as surgical intervention to correct physical abnormalities.

Unfortunately, many practitioners (often family practice physicians or gynecologists) treat depression and anxiety by prescribing the quick-fix antidepressants, with no recommendation for counseling. This type of limited care may help symptoms, but without addressing underlying causes, the chance of getting well and improving interpersonal relationships is poor.

One of the major side effects of some antidepressants is the problem women can have achieving orgasm when taking them. Although some antidepressants (Wellbutrin, for example) have been shown to improve libido, if you are taking antidepressants and are concerned with your low libido, talk to your physician about changing medications or lowering the dose.

Inappropriate Behaviors

Besides the fact that aging sees hormones fade, the body failing, lost libido and the mind beset with confusion and depression, there are certain behaviors that can ruin a relationship even without these other factors coming into play. These behaviors are not usually introduced in the early stages of dating or marriage because, if they were, it's unlikely there would be a commitment made or continued.

Hostile and inappropriate behaviors may be part of a person's psyche, but they are often kept in check. They surface as comfort levels permit. If you or your mate can get away with inappropriate behaviors and they result in the desired effect, they will persist and often get more abusive. They are destructive behaviors that were learned because they usually afford some benefit for those employing them.

Yelling and Screaming

If one of you yells and screams and gets their way, the behavior is reinforced and repeated. If one of you yells and screams and gets ignored or punished, the behavior stops. This is a simplification and is not meant to be a treatise on the various personality disorders that also exhibit behaviors that are inappropriate or negative. Behaviors such as this can make your spouse ill. When not held at bay, these collective negative behaviors lead to many people leaving relationships.

Stop the Nagging

Some call nagging the *marriage killer,* and justifiably so.[18] However, before exploring the nag and its effect on marriage, it needs to be defined. Basically, nagging is really nothing more than asking for something, but it is actually a bit more complicated than that. Nagging is asking for something *more than once over a period of time.* The shorter the time between asking, and the larger the number of times asked results in the more serious cases of nagging. Simply stated, if you ask your mate to do something more than three times over the course of a few minutes, hours, or days, depending upon how important the request is, you have entered the realm of nagging. While nagging is very unpleasant, if you had done what your mate asked at the first request, there would be no nagging. It takes two to *nango.*

Spite can enter into the nagging formula and it makes the problem worse. Either the nagger or the nagged can withhold the desired need from their partner. If the guy or gal wants more sex and is nagging their partner too often, this may result in withholding sex even more and thus lead to the sexless marriage. If the house needs repair or the trash needs to be taken out, the nagged partner, trying to get even with the nagger, may actually neglect these duties as a form of spite. These are childish and destructive behaviors that should be avoided.

Nagging is something most every relationship experiences because it is human nature to put off tasks that are undesirable or those that seem low on the priority list of things that need to be done in a day that is already too short. As universal as nagging may be, it is also risky behavior that can ruin relationships if it is not addressed. When ignored, nagging only gets worse at both ends. The nagger and nagged equally resent each other as time goes by.

Men and women often nag for all the same reasons: having a partner who is chronically late, is messy, talks over the TV, and watches shows he/she doesn't like. They want their partner to do things for them, go places, or do a whole host of things—you can add to the list. For women, the nagging is more likely for getting things, or getting things done, while men usually nag for sex. With women usually being responsible for the home, they often need their men to do chores and fix things around the house. Men might be doing other important things when being nagged, like watching a significant ball game that can't be interrupted.

A terrible dynamic that results in a great deal of toxic nagging is more likely seen with incompatible personality types. An organized, obsessive, on-time kind of person, coupled with a laid back, or lazy, last-minute kind of person results in frustration, arguments, and animosity in each episode of nagging that takes place.

Nagging can become so annoying that soon you argue about nagging and forget the original requests being made. If excessive nagging isn't resolved, your life will be frustrating and filled with resentment.

The first step to resolve nagging is to consider that neither party means harm. The nagger has to realize that she/he is not being ignored out of malice and the nagged has to realize that her/his mate is not making unwarranted pleas. Yes, the dripping faucet needs to be fixed, the trash has to be taken out, and yes, he/she would really like to make love because it feels good even if you don't think so.

Life is all about compromise. If you don't want to be nagged, get off your butt and fulfill the request in a timely manner. *Just do it.* Ignoring your partner is hurtful, disrespectful, and more important; it's very costly when you end up in divorce court. If you truly feel exhausted after a long day and can't satisfy the request immediately, make your case known. Then be specific about when you will comply, and do it as promised.

If you seem to be nagging all the time, recognize that you are probably part of the problem, too. Maybe you're too compulsive about getting things done. Maybe you missed the point that your mate has to unwind after a hard day at work.

Try to communicate in a positive manner by asking when your partner can get the job done and when you should remind them again if they don't act on the request. Now they have agreed on the time to comply and have even accepted a time to be reminded if they weren't compliant.

For some, asking a few times and then just avoiding future requests may work out fine. The partner may make the assumption that their mate is never going to be compliant over certain issues. As long as the issue isn't too big, this may make sense.

The funny thing about life is that, if you were courting, you'd be very careful to honor every request made by your mate in a timely fashion. It's only after complacency enters the relationship that nagging rears its ugly head.

Those involved in excessive nagging are the children who refuse to grow up—the Peter and Patti Pan syndrome.

Is it really true that women nag to get things done and men nag to get sex? Nagging seems to be the consequence of attempting to be heard in an ungracious way. Requests to get things done, and to be at one with your spouse, start as sweet requests. Unless energy is infused into the holy union, it will end unpleasantly.

When the marital garden has not been tended (listening, appreciation, kindness), it slowly degenerates into an abandoned lot full of weeds—weeds that are usually unceremoniously carted out to the trash and dumped. Then the men and women gardeners move upward to a better garden—a new partner who is curious rather than judgmental, acknowledges all that is said and done, and nary a cloud emerges until the garden is in another storm.

The Familiarity Issue

There is also the familiarity issue, the steak-every-night phenomenon where even things that are great can get old after a while. The same mate, the same routine of foreplay, the same position, can and does become old for many. It takes hard work to keep it new, but if you neglect this effort, you only increase your chance for a sexless marriage, with all the attendant consequences. Here are some ideas for keeping it fresh.

- Change positions. One of the easiest things to do is change positions for having sex.

- Sex toys are ways to enliven your sexual encounters.

- Do things together. Some of the best remedies for (WSS) Withholding Sex Syndrome and NPS (Neglected Partner Syndrome) do not take place in the bed at all.

- Work with each other on fantasies that are harmless. If a partner *refusing you* is a turn on, or if there is a *rape fantasy,* set the parameters to make sure no one gets hurt. This also applies to bondage and any dominatrix fantasies. As long as you both agree, trying new things can be fun—or can inform you of what you don't enjoy.

- Undress your partner. Sounds silly, but how many of you begin your sex ritual the same way every time? You hop into bed, get under the covers, and begin whatever activity you have generally started with for the past twenty years. When was the last time you started to be affectionate in the living room or kitchen, began undressing your partner and then moved to the bedroom? If you answered, "yesterday," you are doing it right. If you can't remember the last time you undressed each other, you are probably suffering from familiarity and boring sex.

Financial Matters

Some say that money is the number-one problem in relationships and the number-one reason for divorce.[19]

This book is not meant to be a treatise on finance, nor are any remedies proposed to increase your net worth. However, there are many common-sense ways to combat the effects of financial problems. Simple things like don't try to live up to the mythical Joneses; save for a rainy day; stop buying everything you see; stop buying on credit.

Everyone knows these things to be true. The real problem is the actual behavior with regards to financial matters. Even more conflicting is when you know these things, and your mate does not follow sensible financial dictates.

If there are financial problems causing constant bickering, it's time to seek out financial counseling (not the psychological marriage type). Too many couples don't plan well for the future, and as the future approaches, tremendous pressures come to bear on them.

If you are married to a spendthrift, a compulsive shopper, or someone who must have the best of every modern convenience, and you don't have the means to make such purchases, you have a serious problem. Sadly, many are blind to these traits, even if they'd always been part of their mate's persona ever since they met. Was "love is blind" the reason you never saw your mate's failings? Are both of you irresponsible, fiscally speaking?

It's not easy to change behaviors so embedded. Sometimes it takes a bankruptcy or two to learn. The smart ones wake up on their own once they recognize how financial problems cause tremendous stress and eat at their relationships. For others, prodding by a concerned mate to get the appropriate financial counseling may be needed.

There are still others who, while fiscally responsible, never seem to make ends meet. Perhaps they are stuck in jobs that lead nowhere, they didn't plan for the true costs of raising children, or they've had misfortunes that have kept them out of work. Remedies may not be simple, but even in these situations, talking to financial counselors should provide some plan for relief.

Infidelity

Infidelity is often the end stage of a marriage. This is not to say that there aren't many couples who are able to recover from adulterous affairs and go on to lead happy and healthy relationships. If the couple really wants to reconcile, it usually takes much healing over an extended period of time, along with the help of a qualified therapist.

Questions like, "Can I ever trust again," often plague the aggrieved and may never fade away without a great effort on the part of the adulterer to heal his or her mate through reassurance and deed. The success or failure of reconciliation may have much to do with the many circumstances of the affair. The reasons for reconciliation, such as the realization that divorce has deep social and financial consequences, may suddenly look good, especially if the third party jumps ship. Of course, if those are the only reasons to come back, it would do both parties well to either enter serious counseling to resolve the issues that pulled them apart in the first place, or follow through with divorce.

Infidelity has tremendous consequences for all involved, including the children and the extended family. It is usually not thought out, rather it is acted out on the basis of frustration with the current relationship, or out of lustful intentions. It would be best for those frustrated in their relationships to seek help before falling into the abyss of betrayal. It would be best to look at all of the many issues described in this book and work on making them better before they become unbearable, to make the chances of infidelity or divorce remote.

Affection and Kindness

Sex without affection and kindness is primal and lacks the truest sense of passion and compassion. While primal is what some men and women want, it is not the basis of a sound relationship. If, instead, there is an abundance of affection and kindness and physical health, it's difficult to have a sexless marriage.

You may start with such words of endearment as, "I love you." "You make me so happy when you do that." "I love when you . . ." "You look beautiful/ handsome in that . . ." Notice the little things and acknowledge them. Did he bring you the wrong kind of flowers? Try to appreciate that he brought you flowers at all. Try to appreciate and not criticize. Is there a kind word instead of a hurtful one? Is there dinner on the table? Compliment the cook, even if it isn't perfect. The old adage about catching flies with honey is true. When you show kindness, appreciation, and affection in your words and deeds, you show love.

Besides the kindness and affection of the spoken word, being touchy-feely does wonders for relationships. Hold hands. Rub your mate's shoulders, or feet. Touch his/her arm when you talk. Brush the hair out of her eyes when you gaze into them in conversation. Run your mate a hot bath after a hard day.

Keep It Fresh

To avoid the sexless marriage, keep it fresh with words and deeds. Little things keep your relationship fresh—you didn't go from affectionate to neglectful overnight, but you can begin the comeback immediately.

Ask any divorced person you know. Chances are their ex never used to rub their shoulders, hold their hand, or do any of the usual affectionate physical things that bond couples.

While most people welcome affection, there are reasons beside infidelity that could cause someone to shun endearment. A common fear comes from a mate who is either impotent or frigid. Affection, they might reason, could lead to the bedroom, and that's the last place they want to go when sex is not in the cards for them. This is a serious problem and one that many people avoid discussing out of embarrassment. Here again, the stronger of the two will have to start the dialog and push to learn the reasons why the thrill is gone.

You have to be ready for any and all answers that might come your way. If there is another lover, you don't want to be left in the cold or living a frustrated life without sex. It's better to find out now. If it's a psychological or physical issue keeping your mate from affection due to fear of the bedroom, they may welcome that you were able to start the discussion. Don't be surprised if there is resistance, since a low libido is not a great motivator for getting help in having sex if the partner no longer has any desire for sex.

Start the affection renewal program slowly, and see where it takes you. There may be no need to have that embarrassing discussion or see a therapist if all it takes is a little spark to get the juices flowing again. If you begin with words of endearment for a few weeks and follow up with physical signs of affection, you should see some reciprocation. If reciprocation is forthcoming, go with the flow. Don't be afraid to initiate more advanced physical connection, but don't jump right to sex unless your partner indicates that's where they want to go. Usually a back rub, a foot rub, or just watching television curled up together can do wonders. Little kisses on the cheek for a week can move toward the lips. It may sound juvenile, but if your relationship is in trouble, you need to have a plan with the goal of stimulating the memories that first brought you together. This can be the beginning of *happily ever after*.

Summing Up

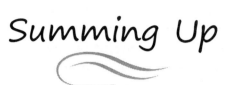

The Six Reasons for Sexual Decline—A Review

These have all been discussed, along with their remedies, throughout the book, but it is appropriate to briefly review them here.

1. Personal issues

2. Behavioral issues

3. Physical issues

4. Psychological issues

5. Hormonal issues

6. A combination of two or more of these issues (the most common problem)

Couples need to be self-aware and rigorously honest to ferret out anything related to these issues that they need to address, or they are unlikely to find success.

Using the traditional path of marriage counseling for sexual problems in the relationship when one or the other partner doesn't have functioning sex organs (a physical/hormonal issue), or has no libido (a psychological/physical/hormonal issue), usually proves to be an exercise in frustration. If one or both are sexually desirous, but no longer interested in their mate (a personal issue), no amount of hormones or counseling will help unless they can resolve this personal issue to regain a whole marriage.

Personal issues of motivation and self-esteem can result in physical decline. If nutrition, diet, and daily exercise have been neglected to the point of developing a myriad of physical and health-related problems, then the appropriate diet, supplementation, and physical activity need to be considered. Taking care of yourself through proper diet and exercise is a most important factor when considering physical issues that can affect your sexual prowess.

The sexless marriage may have one or a multitude of causes and they are often so interconnected that they make the search for answers difficult. If you ever expect to get the appropriate treatment, the importance of receiving the proper diagnosis cannot be overemphasized. The appropriate treatment may not be the standard mainstream approach that has failed so many in years past. New solutions that begin with a blood test may change your life. Yes, a blood test to see if your hormones are in balance. Being so intimately related to every other cause of the sexless marriage, neglecting analysis of your hormones makes finding an appropriate solution remote.

There is always the option to remain in the sexless marriage if it is acceptable to both parties, but if not, a solution can often be found. However, this can only be accomplished by evaluating the six causes and determining which define your situation.

A major symptom of an unhappy relationship is when sex is no longer an important component of the experience if one or both of the partners still wants to engage. The topic of sexless marriage is often so taboo that it is neither discussed nor treated. The end result of this is living in frustration, finding other outlets, or dissolving the relationship.

When asking people whether they still had a desire for sex, and/or were able to function (for men, the ability to achieve/maintain an erection and engage in sex comfortably, and for women, the ability to engage in sex comfortably and climax) their answers were shockingly negative. There are too many married couples living in the same house as roommates.

Many learn to just cope with the sexless marriage even as the relationship deteriorates to the point of being meaningless. If both parties are content with the sex situation, there is no problem other than they may be missing out on a most enjoyable and important bonding experience. If both parties have lost interest and neither one cares, or if sex was never important to them, they are a good match. However, if one or both parties of a sexless marriage want to continue having meaningful sexual relations, then something should be done.

Most couples don't know where to start or who to see to get the help they need to fix the problems associated with a sexless marriage. For those who want to keep their relationship thriving, not just surviving, this book provides you with an opportunity to identify the root causes and fix them with methods that are not all considered mainstream. The journey is not easy. There is no quick-fix for a marriage that has been neglected.

In the final analysis, life is short and offers many bittersweet experiences. Traversing life's joys and sorrows (to teach us grace and wisdom) with a partner makes the trip that much more enjoyable, exciting, tolerable, and worthwhile. Add to the formula, sex, orgasm with your lover, and the drive that has kept the species propagating from the beginning of time, and you have one of life's most beautiful pleasures. Going through this short life with a curious and cooperative partner can make sexuality a profoundly pleasant bonding experience, as well as a highly helpful one in terms of personal growth because this someone knows you better, in all realms, than anyone else.

Yet, with the wrong partner, the relationship can be profoundly unpleasant, frustrating, and destructive. By the time it has become sexless, too many crossroads have been reached, and most partners end up feeling unloved, unappreciated, and unacknowledged, resulting in too many arguments and too many hurtful comments. Nevertheless, by using patience and knowledge, and providing you still like each other, you may find that a return to your former sexual life is possible.

If you find yourself wanting more of what a good life has to offer—and you should—it's time to take charge and make the necessary adjustments to bring joy and fulfillment, complete with the desire to be a sexual couple, back into your marriage. Destiny is part fate and part the choices you make. Don't ever think you can't change your world. Just make sure it's for the better.

Endnotes

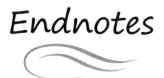

Chapter 2. The Problem

1. Deveny, K. "No Sex, Please, We're Married." *Newsweek*. June 30, 2003.

2. Smith, TW. "American Sexual Behavior: Trends, Socio-Demographic Differences, and Risk Behavior." *National Opinion Research Center*. University of Chicago, April 2003.

3. Stoppler, MC. "Puberty." *MedicineNet.com:* May 4, 2012.

4. Michaels, N. "Sexual Incompatibility in the Divorce Court." *The Modern Law Review*. Vol.29, p 196. Article first published online: Jan. 18, 2011, onlinelibrary. wiley.com.

5. Tavernise, S, Gebeloff, R. "Once Rare in Rural America, Divorce is Changing the Face of Its Families." *The New York Times*. March 23, 2011, A18.

6. Barna Research Group Survey. "Morality Continues to Decay." October 2003, Posted Barna Update, November 2003, www.barna.org.

Chapter 3. Understanding The Forces of Attraction

1. Rako, S. The Hormone of Desire: The Truth about Testosterone, Sexuality, and Menopause. New York, NY: Crown Publishing Group, 1999.

2. Kruger, TH, et al. "Orgasm Induced Prolactin Secretion: Feedback Control of Sex Drive." *Neuroscience Behavioral Review*. 26:1. Jan 2002, 32–44.

Chapter 5. All About Women—Female Sexuality

1. Fuchs, A.R, et al. "Effect of Distention of Uterus and Vagina on Uterine Motility and Oxytocin Release in Puerperal Rabbits." *Acta Endocrinology*. 50:2. October 1965, 239–248.

2. Hertoghe, T. *Passion Sex and Long Life—The Incredible Oxytocin Adventure*. Luxemburg: International Medical Books/Archimedial, January 2010.

3. Freud, S. "The Question of Lay Analysis." 1926e, 212.

4. Freud, S. "The Infantile Genital Organization (an interpolation into theory of sexuality)." (1923e), SE, 20, 141–145.

5. Thompson, NL. "Marie Bonaparte's Theory of Female Sexuality: Fantasy and Biology." *American Imago*. 60:3. Fall 2003, 343–378.

6. Wallen, K,. Lloyd, EA.. "Female Sexual Arousal: Genital Anatomy and Orgasm in Intercourse." *Hormones and Behavior*. 59:5, May 2011, 780–792.

7. Kinsey, AC. *Sexual Behavior in the Human Female*. IN: Indiana University Press, 1953, 575.

8. Masters, W, Johnson, V. *Human Sexual Response,* 1st edition. Toronto, CAN; New York, NY: Bantam Books, 1966.

9. National Survey of Sexual Health and Behavior, Indiana University Center for Sexual Health Promotion," *The Journal of Sexual Medicine* 7:s5, Oct. 2010, 243–373.

10. Grafenberg, E. "The Role of Urethra in Female Orgasm." *The International Journal of Sexology*. 3:3, 1950, 145–148.

11. Activella Homepage, www.activella.com

12. Drugs.com. "Drugs A to Z—Activella—Side Effects." http://www.drugs.com/sfx/activella-side-effects.html

13. Flaherty, JA., Davis, JM., Janicak, PG. *Psychiatry: Diagnosis & Therapy. A Lange Clinical Manual*. Chicago, IL: Appleton and Lange, Northwestern University, 1993, 217.

14. Comfort, A. *The Joy of Sex: Fully Revised and Completely Updated for the 21st Century*. Revised edition. New York, NY: Crown Publishers, October 29, 2002.

Chapter 6. Women and Their Hormones

1. Fournier, A. Berrino, F. Clavel-Chapelon, F. "Unequal Risks for Breast Cancer Associated With Different Hormone Replacement Therapies: Results From The E3N Cohort Study." *Breast Cancer Research and Treatment*. January 2008, 1071, 103–111.

2. Easteal, PW. "Women and Crime: Premenstrual Issues, Australian Institute of Criminology." *Trends and Issues in Crime and Criminal Justice*. 3, April 1991, 1–9.

3. Women's Health Initiative Study. "The Estrogen-Plus Progestin Study." *National Institutes of Health,* July 2, 2002. www.nhlbi.nih.gov/whi/estro_pro.htm

4. Ibid.

5. Chou, WC, et al. "Biomonitoring of Bisphenol A Concentrations in Maternal and Umbilical Cord Blood in Regard to Birth Outcomes and Adipokine Expression: A Birth Cohort Study In Taiwan." *Environmental Health*. 10:94, Nov. 3, 2011; electronic version: www.ehjournal.net/content/10/1/94

6. Campbell, TC, Campbell, TM. The China Study: Startling Implications for Diet, Weight Loss, and Long term Health. Dallas, TX: BenBella Books, January 2005.

7. Gaby, A. Preventing and Reversing Osteoporosis: What You Can Do About Bone Loss—A Leading Expert's Natural Approach to Increasing Bone Mass. New York, NY: Three Rivers Press, 1994.

8. Pfeiffer, CC. Dr. Carl Pfeiffer's Update Fact/Book on Zinc and Other Micro-Nutrients. New Haven, CT: Keats Publishing, 1978.

9. Gaby, A. Preventing and Reversing Osteoporosis: What You Can Do About Bone Loss—A Leading Expert's Natural Approach to Increasing Bone Mass. New York, NY: Three Rivers Press, 1994.

10. Labrie,.F, Acher, D, Bouchard, C, et al. "High Internal Consistency and Efficiency of Intravaginal DHEA for Vaginal Atrophy." *Gynecological Endocrinology.* 2010, 26: 524–532.

11. de la Monte, SM, Wands, JR. "Alzheimer's Disease Is Type Three Diabetes—Evidence Reviewed." *Journal of Diabetes Science and Technology.* 2:6, November 2008, 1101–1113; online: http://www.ncbi.nlm.nih.gov/pmc/articles/PMC 2769828/

12. Hornsby, PJ. "Biosynthesis of DHEAS by Human Adrenal Cortex and Its Age Related Decline." *Annals of the New York Academy of Sciences.* December 1995, 29–46.

13. Hertoghe, T. *Passion, Sex and Long Life—The Incredible Oxytocin Adventure.* Windhof, Luxenburg: International Medical Books, 2010.

14. Wolf, S. *Worst Pills, Best Pills News.* 19:11, November 2013, 2.

15. Carome, M. *Worst Pills, Best Pills News.* 20:11, June 2014, 1.

Chapter 7. All About Men—Male Sexuality

1. R. Shabsigh, et al. "Drivers and Barriers to Seeking Treatment for Erectile Dysfunction: A Comparison of Six Countries," *BJUI International,* 94, (2004) 1055-1065, Wiley online library: www.onlinelibrarywiley.com/doi/10.1111/j.1464-410x .2004.05104.x/pdf

2. Sexual Health Inventory for Men (SHIM), http://www.njurology.com/ _ forms/shim.pdf

3. Feldman, HA, et al. "Impotence and Its Medical and Psychosocial Correlates: Results of The Massachusetts Male Aging Study," *Journal of Urology* 151:1 (Jan 1994) 54-61.

4. Padma-Nathan, H. "Sidenafil Citrate (Viagra) Treatment for Erectile Dysfunction: An Update Profile of Response and Effectiveness," *International Journal of Impotence Research* 18 (2006) 423-431. Doi:10.1038/sj.ijir.3901492; published online 29 June 2006.

5. Pfizer/Viagra website: http://www.pfizer.com/files/products/uspi_viagra.pdf

6. Cohen, ED. "Some Tips on Overcoming Sexual Performance Anxiety." *Psychology Today*. May 28, 2011.

7. Klotz, L. "How (Not) To Communicate New Scientific Information: A Memoir of the Famous Brindley Lecture." *BJUI International* 96:7, November 2005, 956–957.

8. Waldinger, MD, et al. "Original Research-Ejaculation Disorders: A Multinational Population Survey of Intravaginal Ejaculatory Latency Time." *The Journal of Sexual Medicine*. 2:4. July 2005, 492–497.

9. Corty, E, Guardiani, J. "Good Sexual Intercourse Lasts Minutes, Not Hours, Therapists Say." *Penn State, Science Daily*. April 2008.

10. Ignarro, LJ, et al. "Endothelium-Derived Relaxing Factor Produced and Released From Artery and Vein Is Nitric Oxide." *Proceedings of the National Academy of Science*. 84:9, 1987, 9265–9269.

11. "L-arginine: MedlinePlus Supplements" *National Library of Medicine*, www.nlm.nih.gov/medlineplus/druginfo/natural/875.html.

12. Campbell, B, La Bounty, PM, Roberts, M. "The Ergogenic Potential of Arginine." *Journal of the International Society of Sports Nutrition*. 1, 2004, 35–38.

13. Siegel, AL. *Urology*. 84 (1): July 2014, 1–7. doi: 10.1016/j.urology.2014.03.016. Epub May 10, 2014.

14. Hennenfent, B. *Surviving Prostate Cancer Without Surgery*. Roseville, IL: Roseville Books, December 21, 2009.

15. Early Detection of Prostate Cancer: AUA Guideline, *American Urological Association*. http://www.auanet.org/education/guidelines/prostate-cancer-detection.cfm

16. Feldman, HA.. "Age Trends in the Level of Serum Testosterone and Other Hormones In Middle-Age Men: Longitudinal Results From The Massachusetts Male Aging Study." *The Journal of Clinical Endocrinology & Metabolism*. 87:2. February 2002, 589–598.

17. Marsh, JD, et al. "Androgen Receptors Mediate Hypertrophy in Cardiac Myocytes," *Circulation: American Heart Association Journals* 98:3 (1998) 256–261.

18. Shippen, E, Fryer, W. The Testosterone Syndrome: The Critical Factor for Energy, Health, and Sexuality—Reversing the Male Menopause. New York, NY: M. Evans and Company, 1998.

19. Song, Y, Chavarro, Y, Cao, Y, et al. "Whole Milk Intake Is Associated with Prostate-Cancer-Specific Mortality among U.S. Male Physicians." *The Journal of Nutrition*, doi:10.3945/jn.112.168484. December 19, 2012.

20. Bhuiyan, M, Li, Y, Banerjee, S, et al. "Down-regulation of Androgen Receptor by 3,3'-diindolylmethane Contributes to Inhibition of Cell Proliferation and Induction of Apoptosis in Both Hormine-sensitive LNCaP and Insensitive C4-2B Prostate Cancer Cells." *Cancer Research*. 66(20):10064–10072. October, 2006.

21. McPartland, JM, Pruitt, PL. "Benign Prostatic Hyperplasia Treated with Saw Palmetto: A Literature Search and an Experimental Case Study." *The Journal of the American Osteopathic Association*. 100:2. February 1, 2000, 89–96.

22. Shrivastava, A, Gupta, VB. "Various Treatment Options for Benign Prostatic Hypertrophy: A Current Update." *Journal of Mid-Life Health*. 3:1, Jan–June 2012, 10–19.

23. MedlinePlus. Saw Palmetto, online reference: http://www.nlm.nih.gov/medlineplus/druginfo/natural/971.html

Chapter 8. Testosterone

1. Nussey, S, Whitehead, S. *Endocrinology: An Integrated Approach*. Oxford, Great Britain: Bios Scientific Publishers, 2001.

2. Tanriverdi, F, et al. "High Risk of Hypopituitarism after Traumatic Brain Injury: A Prospective Investigation of Anterior Pituitary Function in Acute Phase and 12 Months after Trauma." *The Journal of Clinical Endocrinology & Metabolism*. 91:6, June 2006.

3. Xue, Q. "The Frailty Syndrome: Definition and Natural History." *Clinics in Geriatric Medicine*. 27:1 February 2011. 1–15.

4. Stanworth, RD, Jones, TH. "Testosterone for the Aging Male; Current Evidence and Recommended Practice." *Clinical Interventions in Aging*. 3:1. March, 2008, 25–44.

5. Pugh, PJ, et al. "Testosterone: a Natural Tonic for the Failing Heart?" *QJM, Oxford Journals*. 93:10, 2000, 689–694.

6. Fainaru-Wada, M, Williams, L. "The Truth: Barry Bonds and Steroids." *Sports Illustrated*. March 13, 2006.

7. Fahim, MS, et al. "Effect of Panax Ginseng on Testosterone Level and Prostate in Male Rats." *Archives of Andrology*. 8:4, June 1982, 261–263.

8. Wu, H, et al. "Chemical and Pharmacological Investigations of Epimedium Species: A Survey." *Progress in Drug Research*. 60, 2003, 1–57.

9. Gonzales, GF, et al., "Effect of Lepidium Meyenii (Maca), A Root With Aphrodisiac and Fertility Enhancing Properties, On Serum Reproductive Hormone Levels in Adult Healthy Men," *Journal of Endocrinology* 176 (January, 1, 2003) 163–168.

10. Talbott, SM, et al. "Effect of Tongkat Ali on Stress Hormones and Psychological Mood State in Moderately Stressed Subjects." *Journal of the International Society of Sports Nutrition*. 10:28. May 26, 2013.

11. Netter, A, Hartoma, R, Nahoul, K. "Effect of Zinc Administration on Plasma Testosterone, Dihydrotestosterone, and Sperm Count." *Archives of Andrology*. 7:1, August 1981, 69–73.

12. Pilz, S, et al. "Effect of Vitamin D Supplementation on Testosterone Levels In Men." *Hormone and Metabolic Research*. 43:3, March 2011, 223–225.

13. Caronia, L. "Testosterone Decreases After Ingestion of Sugar (Glucose)." Study presented at The Endocrine Society, May 20, 2010.

14. Meta, PH, Joseph RA. "Testosterone and Cortisol Jointly Regulate Dominance: Evidence for a Dual-Hormone Hypothesis." *Hormone Behavior.* 58:5, November 2010, 898–906.

15. Hamalainen, E, et al. "Diet and Serum Sex Hormones in Healthy Men." *Journal of Steroid Biochemistry.* 20:1, January 1984, 459–464.

16. Melville, NA. "Low Testosterone Levels Can Improve With Weight Loss, Exercise." *The Endocrine Society 94th Annual Meeting,* presented June 25, 2012.

17. Roden, EL, Morgentaler, A. "Medical Progress: Risks of Testosterone-Replacement Therapy and Recommendations for Monitoring." *The New England Journal of Medicine.* 350, Jan 2004, 482–492.

18. Pechersky, AV, et al. "Androgen Administration in Middle-Aged and Aging Men: Effects of Oral Testosterone Undecanoate on Dihydrotestosterone, Oestradiol and Prostate Volume." *International Journal of Andrology.* 2:2 April 2002, 119–125.

19. Hamilton, J. "Most Plastics Leach Hormone-Like Substances." *NPR New, Science Online:* http://www.npr.org/2011/03/02/134196209/study-most-plastics-leach-hormone-like-chemicals, March 2, 2011.

20. Hertoghe, T. *The Hormone Handbook—The Keys to Safe Hormone Therapies: How to Do it and How to Solve Therapy Problems.* Windhof, Luxemburg: SA International Medical Books, 2010, 216.

21. Morgentaler, A. *Testosterone for Life: Recharge Your Vitality, Sex Drive, Muscle Mass, and Overall Health.* New York, NY: McGraw-Hill, October, 2008.

Chapter 9. Physical Issues

1. Nusbaum, MRH, et al. "Chronic Illness and Sexual Functioning." *American Family Physician.* 67:2, January, 15, 2003, 347.

2. Jackson, G, et al. "Erectile Dysfunction and Coronary Artery Disease Prediction: Evidence-Based Guidance and Consensus." *International Journal of Clinical Practice.* 64:7, June 2010, 848–857.

3. Nusbaum, MRH, et al. "Chronic Illness and Sexual Functioning." *American Family Physician.* 67:2, January, 15, 2003, 352.

4. Hamilton, A.B. "Psychological Aspects of Ovarian Cancer." *Cancer Investigation.* 17, 1999, 335–341.

5. Nusbaum, MRH, et al. *Ibid,* 352.

6. Kinsey, AC, et al. *Sexual Behavior in the Human Female.* Philadelphia, PA: W.B. Saunders Company, 1953.

Chapter 10. Psychological Issues

1. Seidman, SN, Roose, SP. "The Relationship Between Depression and Erectile Dysfunction." *Current Psychiatry Reports.* 2, 2000, 201–205.

2. Masters, WH, Johnson, VE. *Human Sexual Response,* (Toronto, CAN, New York, NY: Bantam Books, 1966.

3. "Types of HSDD in women," www.HSDDonline.com/types-of-hsdd.html

4. Health and Education Publications, National Institute of Mental Health." *National Institute of Health online:* http://www.nimh.nih.gov/health/publications/ the-numbers-count-mental-disorders-in-america/index.shtml

5. Wurtman, JJ. "Depression and Weight Gain: The Serotonin Connection." *Journal of Affective Disorder.* 29:2–3, Oct-Nov 1993, 183–192.

Chapter 11. Personal and Behavioral Issues

1. Nusbaum, MRH, et al. "Chronic Illness and Sexual Functioning." *American Family Physician.* 67:2, January, 15, 2003, p. 352.

2. Klunsmann, D. "Sexual Motivation and The Durations of Partnership," *Archives of Sexual Behavior* 31:3, July 2002, 275–287.

3. Bergner, D. "Unexcited? There May Be A Pill for That." *New York Times Magazine,* May 22, 2013.

4. Perel, E. *Mating In Captivity: Unlocking Erotic Intelligence.* New York, NY: HarperCollins, 2006.

5. Gray, E. "Does Monogamy Cause Female Sexual Dysfunction—And Could A Pill Be The Answer?" *The Huffington Post.* 5/24/2013.

6. Meyer, C. "Why The Passive Aggressive Woman Withholds Sex." *Divorce Support:* http://divorcesupport.about.com/od/isdivorcethesolution/u/family_issues.htm.

7. Kreger, R. "Stop Walking on Egg Shells." *Psychology Today.* February 26, 2012.

8. Williams, JE, et al. "Effects of an Angry Temperament on Coronary Heart Disease Risk." *American Journal of Epidemiology.* 154:3, 2001, 230–235.

9. Greenberg, M. "Why We Gain Weight When We're Stressed—And How Not To." *Psychology Today.* August 28, 2013.

10. De Sousa, A, Sonavane, S, Mehta, J. "Psychological Aspects of Prostate Cancer." *Prostate Cancer and Prostatic Diseases.* 15:2, 2012, 120–127.

11. Ben-Zeev, A. "Why Make-Up Sex and Breakup Sex Are So Good." *Psychology Today, In The Name of Love.* February 10, 2013.

12. Hendrix, H. *Getting the Love You Want: A Guide for Couples.* New York, NY: Henry Holt and Company, 1988.

13. FastStats. "Life Expectancy." Centers for Disease Control and Prevention: http://www.cdc.gov/nchs/fastats/lifepec.htm.

14. Rosen, RC, Lane, RM, Menza, M. "Effects of SSRIs on Sexual Function: A Critical Review." *Journal of Clinical Psychopharmacology.* 19:1 February 1999, 67–85.

15. Arafa, M, Shamloul, R. "A Randomized Study Examining The Effect of 3 SSRI on Premature Ejaculation Using A Validated Questionnaire." *Journal of Therapeutics and Clinical Risk Management.* 3:4, August 2007, 527–531.

16. "Drugs that May Cause Impotence." *National Library of Medicine.* www.nlm. nih.gov/medlineplus/ency/article/ 004024.html.

17. FDA. "Menopause and Hormones." July 26, 2013: www.fda.gov/forconsumers/byaudience/forwomen/ucm118624.htm

18. Bernstein, E. "Meet the Marriage Killer." *The Wall Street Journal.* January 25, 2012.

19. McGraw, PC. "Money: Financial and Marital Harmony." Dr. Phil online: http://www.drphil.com/articles/article/32

Recommended Reading

Integrative Physicians

Golan, Ralph. *Optimal Wellness: Where Mainstream and Alternative Medicine Meet.* New York, NY: Ballantine Books, 1995.

Hertoghe, Thierry. *The Hormone Solution—Stay Younger Longer with Natural Hormone and Nutritional Therapies.* New York, NY: Three Rivers Press, 2002.

Hertoghe, Thierry. *The Hormone Handbook—The Keys to Safe Hormone Therapies: How to Do it and How to Solve Therapy Problems.* Windhof, Luxemburg: SA International Medical Books, 2010.

Lichten, Edward. *Textbook of Bio-Identical Hormones.* Fort Lauderdale, FL: Foundation for Anti-Aging Research, 2007.

Platt, Michael. *The Miracle of Bio-Identical Hormones—How I Lost My Fatigue–Hot Flashes–ADHA-ADD–Fibromyalgia–PMS–Osteoporosis– Weight–Sexual Dysfuction–Anger–Migraines.* Rancho Mirage, CA: Clancy Lane Publishing, 2007.

Reiss, Uzzi, Reiss-Gendell, Yfat. *The Natural Superwoman—The Scientifically Backed Program for Feeling Great, Looking Younger, and Enjoying Amazing Energy at Any Age.* New York, NY: Avery, 2007.

Resources

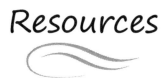

Associations

American Association of Naturopathic Physicians
Phone: 866-538-2267
Website: www.naturopathic.org

American College for Advancement in Medicine (ACAM)
Phone: 888-439-6891
Website: www.acamnet.org

International College of Integrative Medicine
Phone: 419-358-0273
Website: www.icimed.com

Pharmacy Compounding Accreditation Board
Website: http://www.pcab.org

Because custom bio-identical drugs are not mainstream, you may have difficulty locating a local compounding pharmacy. If you can't find a doctor to prescribe compounded remedies, you can contact a compounding pharmacy through the above website and they may be able to direct you to a doctor who can help you.

Once you locate a doctor who understands and prescribes these medications, she/he can recommend a pharmacy that will fill your prescription and mail it to you overnight if necessary.

Dr. Morgan currently works with the following compounding pharmacies and feels comfortable with their preparations.

Jersey Shore Pharmacy
3007 Ocean Heights Avenue
Egg Harbor Township, NJ 08234

Hopewell Pharmacy and Compounding Center
1 West Broad Street
Hopewell, NJ 08525

Natural Supplements/
Alternative Health Resources

The nutritional supplements mentioned in this book are available at health food stores, on the Internet, and even in pharmacies that are getting in on the program as they realize the benefits to be gained. Be a sophisticated consumer. Make sure you do some research to get the best quality, most effective supplements at reasonable prices. Consider that the biggest supplement companies have the most to lose if they are found to have inferior products. As such, they are more inclined to have third-party laboratory analysis done to make sure purity, quality, and quantity are standardized so you get what it says on the bottle.

Male Enhancement Formulas
Agri-ViveIII, Ultra Turbo, and Ultimate Vigor supplied by:
Real Advantage Nutrients, Campbell Douglas, II, M.D.
702 Cathedral Street
Baltimore, MD 21201
Phone: 800-913-2602
Website: http://www.realadvantage nutrients.com

Primal Max supplied by:
Primal Force, Inc., Al Sears M.D.
11905 Southern Blvd.
Royal Palm Beach, FL 33411
Phone: 866-895-8555
Website: htpp://www.primalforce.net

Male™ and Vicariin Virility Formula supplied by:
Tahoma Clinic Dispensary, Jonathan Wright M.D.
6839 Fort Dent Way, Suite 125
Tukwila, WA 98188
Phone: 888-893-6878
Website: htpp://www.tahomadispensary.com

Computer Program

Heart Math—emWave technology made for your computer. The program will teach you how to control your heartbeats with breathing.
Phone: 800-450-9111
Website: http://www.heartmathstore.com/

Index

About the Authors

How do an endodontist and a medical doctor come to write the most explosive book about the genesis of, and cure for, a sexless marriage or sexless relationship? Doctors Fleisher and Foss-Morgan decided to put their knowledge and experience together—his as researcher/ writer of medical and health guides, and hers as a specialist in integrative medicine and bio-identical hormone replacement—to explore a subject deemed so taboo that the usual path of ignoring the problem has resulted in more breakups and more people living in frustrating, unhealthy relationships than all other reasons combined.

Through case studies, the sad story of sexless unions comes to life. There is, however, hope. That hope starts with a series of blood tests, but identifying the problem is just the beginning. Doctors Fleisher and Foss-Morgan demonstrate their expertise in a very readable, concise volume that combines medical, sexual, and relationship advice.

Dr. Fleisher has had the opportunity to treat over 30,000 patients in his career. While his practice was the dental specialty of endodontics, he also writes extensively on aging. As an *Examiner.com* journalist, he writes a column on relationships and Internet dating. He developed and wrote an interactive course, *Bedside Manner: How to Gain Your Patients' Respect, Love and Loyalty,* which he teaches to his residents at Albert Einstein Medical Center in Philadelphia via his website/blog: www.bedsidemanner.info. Dr. Fleisher has authored numerous articles for professional publications, appeared on radio shows across the country discussing how HPV is involved in cervical and oral cancer, and he lectures nationally.

Dr. Morgan was the medical director of the Princeton Longevity Center where she honed her skills on nutritional biochemistry, bio-identical hormone replacement therapy (BHRT), neuropsychiatry, and regeneration of medical illness, utilizing both conventional and complementary medicine.

She also studies with leading endocrinologists in Europe, and is currently the director of the Morgan Center for Integrative Medicine where her practice focuses on bio-identical hormone supplementation and sexual-enhancement therapies for both men and women.

Dr. Morgan has appeared on *CNN*, *Fox News*, and many radio shows, and she frequently lectures to physicians and patients.

CPSIA information can be obtained at www.ICGtesting.com
Printed in the USA
BVOW01s0908280716

457165BV00012B/92/P